D1405850

DR. ISADORE ROSENFELD'S
BREAKTHROUGH
HEALTH

167 Up-to-the-Minute
Medical Discoveries,
Treatments, and Cures
That Can Save Your Life,
**from America's
Most Trusted Doctor!**

BY ISADORE ROSENFELD, M.D.

2004 EDITION

RODALE

Notice

This book is intended as a reference volume only, not as a medical manual. The information given here is designed to help you make informed decisions about your health. It is not intended as a substitute for any treatment that may have been prescribed by your doctor. If you suspect that you have a medical problem, we urge you to seek competent medical help.

Mention of specific companies, organizations, or authorities in this book does not imply endorsement by the author or publisher, nor does mention of specific companies, organizations, or authorities imply that they endorse this book, its author, or the publisher.

Internet addresses and telephone numbers given in this book were accurate at the time it went to press.

© 2004 by Isadore Rosenfeld, M.D.

All rights reserved. No part of this publication may be reproduced or transmitted in any form or by any means, electronic or mechanical, including photocopying, recording, or any other information storage and retrieval system, without the written permission of the publisher.

Printed in the United States of America
Rodale Inc. makes every effort to use acid-free ∞, recycled paper ♻.

Book design by Drew Frantzen

ISBN 1–57954–995–0 hardcover
ISBN 1–57954–900–4 paperback

Distributed to the book trade by St. Martin's Press

2 4 6 8 10 9 7 5 3   hardcover
   4 6 8 10 9 7 5 3   paperback

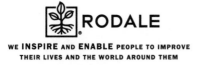

WE **INSPIRE** AND **ENABLE** PEOPLE TO IMPROVE
THEIR LIVES AND THE WORLD AROUND THEM

FOR MORE OF OUR PRODUCTS
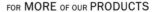
WWW.RODALESTORE.COM
(800) 848-4735

FOR MY CAMILLA—AGAIN. WIFE, MOTHER, GRANNY, FRIEND—AND MY CONTINUING INSPIRATION FOR ALMOST A HALF CENTURY! (SHE WAS ONLY A KID WHEN IT ALL BEGAN.)

CONTENTS

ACKNOWLEDGMENTS

SPECIAL THANKS to my superb editor, Leah Flickinger, for her vital role in the preparation of this book. Intelligent, relentlessly hard-working, perceptive, possessed of great judgment—and fun. I didn't really mind her incessant phone calls and e-mails designed, I know, to make sure we met all the deadlines. She deserves an honorary M.D.!

Special thanks also to my friend and agent Joni Evans who, with her usual perspicacity, has made this book possible. She worked with Leah and me on every stage of the book and her advice was, as usual, indispensable.

The value of a resource such as this book depends on meticulous confirmation of the facts presented. I am very grateful for the help provided me by my publisher, who assigned an extremely knowledgeable fact-checker to this project. Christina Bilheimer has, with great devotion and skill, ascertained the accuracy of the information on these pages.

Finally, I am both grateful and in awe of the genius and work of the many scientists, doctors, and researchers whose findings I have reported in these pages. Hope should spring eternal for the sick because of the dedication of these men and women to the welfare of mankind.

INTRODUCTION

THE EXPLOSION OF MEDICAL KNOWLEDGE from university laboratories, pharmaceutical companies, and other research facilities here
and abroad means that more can be done for you when you're sick
than ever. I've said this many times before, but it bears repeating:
most doctors—even those who keep up-to-date—don't have the time
to share this information with you. So it's really up to you to stay
abreast of what's going on in medicine. In truth, many doctors expect you to do so.

Myriad reports in the media and on the Internet do not usually
interpret new findings or translate them into information that you
can use. That's why I wrote this book. In it, you will read all about
the latest breakthroughs, the cutting edge of medicine, and the most
interesting, important, and practical discoveries for whatever ails
you. I have interpreted and evaluated them for you as if you were my
own patient sitting with me in my office. Here are some examples of
what these pages contain.

- Are you at risk for developing diabetes because other members
  of your family have it, you're overweight, or your blood glucose levels are borderline or slightly elevated? Do you know
  how to reduce that risk?

- Do you know that if you need aspirin but can't take it because it irritates your stomach or makes your ulcer bleed, eradicating a common but silent gastric infection caused by a bacterium can solve your problem?

- Do you think you're too old to bother treating your high cholesterol level? Read what happened to 80- and 90-year-olds who lowered theirs with a statin drug.

- Have you had an angioplasty and become fearful that you may be one of the 30 percent of patients in whom the sleeve that keeps the artery open (the stent) will close up? Read about the new, coated stents in which this happens less often.

- Are you envious of your friends who have followed Atkins-type diets and lost weight, but you're afraid to eat all that saturated fat and cholesterol? Read the latest findings about the safety and efficacy of these diets.

- If there's a strong history of breast cancer in your family, do you know that one of the pills already in your medicine cabinet can protect you against this disease?

- Some of your friends have been getting Botox injections to get rid of facial wrinkles. Are you aware that these injections can also control body odor and reduce migraine or cluster headaches?

- Do you know when not to take the popular antioxidant vitamins C and E—and why not?

- Are you worried because one of your relatives who was ostensibly in good health, without any of the usual risk factors for vascular disease, suddenly had a heart attack at age 50? Do you know about the blood test that indicates vulnerability to heart attacks and strokes even when all other predictive factors are normal?

This book is full of such news items (and many more) that you may not have heard about. I have evaluated all of them for you. I have separated fact from fiction, hype from hope. In each case, I make it clear what I'd advise you to do if you were my own patient.

I plan to continue providing you with this kind of information year after year—you'll never be in the dark again. The table of contents and the index will give you a good idea of the scope of the major medical advances this past year. Refer to the sections that interest you most, but also look at the other chapters. As you scan the table of contents, you'll notice I've organized this book alphabetically by disease or condition, with individual entries devoted to each breakthrough. That's because I want to make it as easy as possible for you to locate the information that's relevant to you. But not every breakthrough in medicine fits neatly into one disease category or another, so I've taken a number of these reports and put them in a slightly different format. Whenever you see the words "What the Doctor Ordered?", you know you'll be reading about something that has implications beyond the scope of the chapter, is especially controversial, or debunks a widespread belief. Is this information what the doctor ordered? Read and find out.

I hope you'll find this book as fascinating to read as I did to research, and that you'll discover something that may help you or someone you care about.

ALCOHOLISM

New Hope for Alcoholics

ACCORDING TO THE NATIONAL INSTITUTES OF HEALTH, 1 in every 13 American adults "abuses alcohol" or is an "alcoholic." (I have never understood the difference between these two groups.) I don't know how those figures were obtained, but there is no question in my mind that more of us than that engage in binge drinking or drink heavily enough on a regular basis to lead to more severe problems. I also suspect that those who have been harmed by alcohol know deep down that they have a problem, or at least a potential one. They may rationalize it to others, but in their heart of hearts they sense that they need help. The tragedy is that they do not always ask for it and when they do, it's not always available or effective.

Here's a simple self-test that can help you recognize a drinking problem. Ask yourself the following four questions.

- Have you ever felt you should cut down on your drinking?

- Do people annoy you when they criticize your drinking?

- Do you ever feel bad or guilty about your drinking?
- Do you need an eye-opener first thing in the morning to steady your nerves or get rid of a hangover?

If you answered yes to even one of these questions, you may have a drinking problem and you should look more closely at the matter, especially if other members of your immediate family have one too.

Although there is no cure for alcoholism, there are steps you can take to cope with it. Look into support groups such as Alcoholics Anonymous (they have helped many problem drinkers). Marital and psychological counseling may be useful. When all else fails, check into a detoxification program. (Unfortunately, some 50 percent of those treated eventually go back to drinking.)

Many problem drinkers look to prescription medications for help with their problem. Three drugs are available:

1. **Antabuse (disulfiram)** makes you so sick if you dare to drink while you're on it that you're terrified to ever booze again. It sounds good on paper, but this medication is not prescribed much anymore—for two reasons. Some of its adverse effects are severe and can harm the alcoholic, especially if he or she has some other significant underlying disease. More commonly, however, having tasted what wrath can befall them if they drink while on Antabuse, most drinkers stay with the booze and avoid the medication. The cure is worse than the disease!

2. **Naltrexone**, originally introduced to control cravings for heroin and other narcotics, was approved by the FDA for keeping people off alcohol once they've quit. However, its reported effectiveness is disputed. One study found it to be of no use at all; another claimed success in one-third to one-half of patients treated. I've found its benefit to be limited among my patients.

3. **Acamprosate** is available in Europe but not yet in the United States. It acts on neurotransmitters in the brain to control the desire to drink. It helps in some cases.

■ HERE'S WHAT'S NEW

Researchers at the University of Texas Health Science Center in San Antonio have discovered that topiramate (marketed as Topamax), an approved antiseizure drug made from a naturally occurring sugar and used to treat epilepsy, appears to be much more effective in helping alcoholics quit drinking than any other drug available. According to their paper, published in the journal *The Lancet*, topiramate works by washing away excess dopamine, a chemical in the brain that enhances the craving for alcohol.

The researchers studied 103 heavy drinkers (men who regularly consumed more than five drinks a day and women who took more than four), all of whom had already tried and failed Alcoholics Anonymous, drug therapy, psychotherapy, and rehabilitation clinics. Fifty-five subjects were given oral topiramate; the remaining 48, a placebo. At the end of the study, 24 percent of those taking the topiramate had abstained completely for 1 month, compared with only 4 percent of the placebo group. Another plus for topiramate was that it improved abnormal liver function caused by alcohol excess in some patients. It also lifted mood and relieved anxiety symptoms.

Topiramate differs from all other antialcohol regimens, whose success is judged by the duration of abstinence. Patients on topiramate do not have to abstain completely. However, if they do continue to drink, they do so less than before. And, 2 drinks are better—and safer—than 10. On all these accounts, the data strongly suggest that topiramate is more effective than either naltrexone or acamprosate.

Long-term use of topiramate by epileptics has shown the drug to be safe in most cases, but you should be aware of some possible complications. If you have glaucoma, this drug can make the condition worse. Topiramate can also interfere with the body's heat-regulating mechanism. Several cases of overheating and dehydration have been reported (mostly in kids being treated for epilepsy). Some questions have also been raised about topiramate's adverse effect on cognition (memory and thinking processes).

Although researchers will likely continue to study this medication, experts are already hailing it as "a major scientific advance in the treatment of alcoholism." In fact, investigators are also evaluating it for the treatment of obesity.

■ THE BOTTOM LINE

Topiramate appears to be more effective than other drugs currently available for treating alcohol addiction. The scientific community is impressed with its results in one well-controlled study and will surely continue to evaluate it. It is already on the market (albeit for another purpose), so if you or a loved one has a severe alcohol problem and other therapies have failed, your doctor can get topiramate for you.

ALZHEIMER'S DISEASE

The Latest News on Prevention

ACCORDING TO OFFICIAL ESTIMATES, about four million Americans have Alzheimer's disease (AD). However, the symptoms of this degenerative brain disorder can be so subtle that many "normal" people who are already in its early stages choose to deny them and go undiagnosed. I can't say I blame them given that, at the moment, there is no really effective treatment for the disease. We used to deny impotence in much the same way. "Impotent? Who, me? Naw. I'm just overworked." Then came Viagra, and suddenly millions of men who had deluded their partners, their doctors, and even themselves into believing they were sexual athletes began lining up for this new prescription. If and when there is a similar breakthrough for Alzheimer's, I predict that the four million number will escalate well into the double-digit millions. As it stands, the aging baby boomers are expected to swell that number to 14 million in the next few years.

■ HERE'S WHAT'S NEW

There is a great deal of interest and research into Alzheimer's at this time. New observations about its risk factors, how it can be predicted, and what can be done to prevent it are frequently in the news. This past year, at least seven large studies reached a number of important conclusions.

Researchers at Rush-Presbyterian/St. Luke's Medical Center in Chicago found that diets rich in saturated fat create a greater risk for Alzheimer's. People who regularly consumed the most saturated fat were found to have a 2.3 times greater risk for Alzheimer's than those whose diets were habitually lowest in saturated fats. (Saturated fats are present mostly in meats and dairy products.)

By the same token, foods high in monounsaturated and polyunsaturated fats decrease the risk. Examples of monounsaturated fats are olive and canola oils. The richest (and healthiest) sources of polyunsaturated fat (omega-3 fatty acids) are fatty fish, as well as plant and vegetable oils rich in alpha-linoleic and linoleic acid (corn and safflower oils). A deficiency of these acids has been implicated in several mental disorders other than Alzheimer's.

High blood pressure, well-documented as a cause of heart attack and stroke, is another risk factor for AD, especially in people over age 75. These findings strengthen the argument for treating elevated blood pressure as vigorously in the elderly as in the young.

An elevated homocysteine level is also a predictor of Alzheimer's disease. Researchers assume, but have not yet proven, that lowering or normalizing homocysteine may make a difference.

We already know that certain genes are associated with a higher incidence of AD. Still, you may have the gene and never develop AD, or not have it and get the disease anyway. However, there is one gene, the apolipoprotein E gene, that does appear to have significant predictive value for AD. Its presence is associated with an almost threefold incidence of the disease, but only in whites, not in African-Americans.

Recent studies refute a long-held belief that antioxidants such as carotenes, vitamins C and E, and a variety of other nutrients protect against AD. Patients taking these supplements do not have a lower incidence of this disorder. However, several studies do emphasize the protective effect of two types of drugs: the statins that lower cholesterol and, as I'll discuss in greater detail starting on page 8, aspirin and other nonsteroidal anti-inflammatory drugs (NSAIDs). However, these medications have no effect if the disease is already present.

The latest research indicates that in postmenopausal women over age 65, estrogen-progesterone replacement therapy actually raises the risk of Alzheimer's disease and induces milder memory loss as well. Earlier studies had already implicated hormone replacement therapy as contributing to heart disease and stroke.

▪ THE BOTTOM LINE

I, personally, am not keen to learn whether I carry the genes that are likely to cause Alzheimer's sometime in the future. What's the point? There is nothing I can do about it except follow the diet I describe above. I do that anyway. Learning that I have a good chance of losing my marbles when I get older simply would take the pleasure out of life while I still have them.

The other measures to prevent AD are to keep your blood pressure normal and your cholesterol down. Statin drugs—the prototype of which is Lipitor (atorvastatin), though there are many others—not only lower high cholesterol, they also appear to have a protective anti-inflammatory effect against AD. Also, the anti-inflammatory properties of NSAIDs, such as Motrin (ibuprofen) and Aleve (naproxen) are believed to delay or prevent AD, although they have no impact on symptoms once the disease has begun. So if you are caring for someone with Alzheimer's, you can use NSAIDs to treat their chronic pain, but it won't help their senile dementia. Also watch out for gastrointestinal bleeding, a common side effect of these drugs, especially in the elderly.

Preserve Your Memory with Anti-Inflammatories

ALTHOUGH SOME DEMENTIA RESEARCH has focused on whether vascular problems such as high blood pressure or high cholesterol levels contribute to Alzheimer's, AD is not a vascular brain disease. It bears no relation to a stroke. In fact, millions of people with normal blood flow to the brain are affected by AD. While the cause of Alzheimer's disease is unclear, inflammation is now believed to play a role. So the latest news about the beneficial effects of anti-inflammatories such as aspirin and NSAIDs on this disorder comes as no surprise.

■ HERE'S WHAT'S NEW

Several studies, from such highly regarded institutions as the University of Washington in Seattle and Johns Hopkins in Baltimore, have shown the effectiveness of NSAIDs in the *prevention* of Alzheimer's. Subjects who took any one of these agents daily for at least 2 years had a 73 percent reduced risk of developing Alzheimer's. Aspirin was also beneficial but not to the same degree. Its daily use was found to reduce the subsequent risk of Alzheimer's by only 13 percent.

■ THE BOTTOM LINE

Taking aspirin should be a no-brainer for most adults who can tolerate it. Given its protective effect against heart attack and stroke, a daily aspirin is usually a good idea, especially for anyone who already suffers from vascular disease or who is still healthy but vulnerable. So discuss it with your doctor. It may not be advisable for people who have bleeding or clotting problems, who take blood thinners, who bleed from time to time from the intestinal tract, or who have asthma.

If you have a family history of Alzheimer's or have been tested for the gene and found to have it, I suggest a daily NSAID for prevention. (Remember, however, that many people who are found to have the gene never develop Alzheimer's—and vice versa.) I believe that enough evidence exists for most people to take an anti-inflammatory at a low dose if their doctor has determined that it is safe for them to do so. Just keep in mind that this measure works only while you're still "with it." NSAIDs won't help once symptoms of Alzheimer's have appeared. However, if you have several risk factors for heart disease or stroke, or already have evidence of either of these vascular diseases, then you should take an aspirin instead of an NSAID. Unfortunately, the combination of the two may cause stomach problems, especially in older people.

DHEA for Alzheimer's? Forget about It!

IF YOU'VE SPENT ANY TIME BROWSING THE INTERNET, you likely are familiar with the "wonder hormone" called dehydroepiandrosterone (DHEA). There are literally hundreds of Web sites, in almost every language, where you can read about this miraculous product. And there's no problem getting as much of it as you want without a prescription. Another big "plus" is that you can pay for it in any currency you happen to have.

DHEA is produced by the adrenal glands that sit atop the kidneys. No one knows for sure what its function really is. Some years ago, it was noted that very early in life the body makes little of it. Then, starting at about age 6, its production is increased and peaks in the mid-twenties. (Men always have a little more than women.) From then on, it's all downhill. By age 75, both sexes have only 20 percent of the DHEA that they did 50 years earlier.

What an opportunity for "health" product entrepreneurs! Never mind trying to figure out why the body makes so much less as we age. That would take too long. Instead, these entrepreneurs act on the assumption that because we have tons of DHEA when we're young and healthy, but by 75 we have very little, taking lots and lots of it as we grow older will help us stay (or become) young. Many thousands of people have fallen for this Internet sales pitch, and DHEA is selling by the carload.

Meanwhile, the FDA does not regulate DHEA, because they do not consider it a drug; instead, they've designated it a "dietary supplement." That can mean trouble for consumers. In a recent analysis of 16 DHEA products on sale in the United States, one was found to contain absolutely none of the hormone; two had only a trace; the DHEA content in the remaining 13 ranged from 69 to 150 percent of what the label claimed!

DHEA does appear to have a beneficial effect in experiments on mice and rats. However, there's a big difference between rodents and people. For starters, these animals produce only 1/10,000 the amount of DHEA that we do.

The results of studies on humans have been mixed—some have been favorable, others have not. So why not just take the hormone? What harm can it do?

As I mentioned previously, we don't really understand what DHEA's function is. It may be simply a waste product of hormonal production. But we do know that it eventually ends up as estrogen and testosterone. (Saddam Hussein might have referred to it as "the mother of all hormones," and the FDA actually calls it the "mother hormone.") Taking extra DHEA means being saddled with more estrogen and testosterone, which may increase the risk of developing hormone-based cancers (of the breast in women and the prostate in men). Maybe I'm too conservative, but that's one important reason why I do not recommend DHEA for *any* patient. And until the FDA begins supervising its production, you're buying a pig in the poke with every bottle you purchase.

■ HERE'S WHAT'S NEW

Acting on the observation that in some studies DHEA did improve memory in older mice, researchers at the University of California at San Francisco evaluated this effect in 58 people with Alzheimer's disease. This was a double-blind study in which half the participants received a placebo. Every patient was tested for thinking and memory function throughout the study. Although after 3 months there was a small but insignificant benefit in the DHEA-treated group, by 6 months there was no major difference between the two groups.

■ THE BOTTOM LINE

The results of this small study do not support using DHEA to improve memory among the elderly. Until more research results are in, I wouldn't recommend the hormone for any reason. There are other, better ways to feel young—exercise and mental stimulation being among the most important.

WHAT THE DOCTOR ORDERED?

WHAT ABOUT GINKGO BILOBA?

■ Ginkgo biloba is a bestselling feel-good herb. Complain about anything, and most complementary medicine enthusiasts will recommend ginkgo. It's a powerful antioxidant that has been used for centuries to treat a host of ailments. In this country, it is especially popular for improving cognition (thinking and memory), and some doctors, especially those with a bent toward alternative medicine, recommend it for people with Alzheimer's disease (AD).

In my book *Dr. Rosenfeld's Guide to Alternative Medicine*, published in 1996, I too, suggested it for this purpose because a study by the New York Institute for Medical Research found evidence of some cognitive improvement in AD patients taking ginkgo. Also, it appeared that this herb increases blood flow to the brain. Since then, the validity of the New York findings has been questioned, and proof of any major benefit from ginkgo is sparse. However, several studies continue to evaluate ginkgo and, who knows, they may show that it does help.

HERE'S WHAT'S NEW

Several healthy patients of mine who don't have even the slightest evidence of AD take ginkgo to improve memory and their "thinking processes." Will this herb help them? Recent studies suggest that it won't. Researchers at Williams College in Massachusetts who received a grant from the National Institutes of Health conducted a well-designed double-blind, randomized, controlled trial to determine whether ginkgo improved memory in 230 physically active and mentally healthy volunteers older than age 60. Half of the subjects took a 40-milligram tablet of ginkgo three times a day; the others were given a placebo. At the end of 6 weeks, all were tested for verbal and nonverbal learning, memory, attention, concentration, and expressive language (finding the right word). There was no difference whatsoever in the performances of the two groups.

As you've read elsewhere in this book, the FDA does not regulate or inspect herbal supplements as it does drugs. As a result, several popular supplements, on which millions of Americans pin their hopes and spend their money, are not what they are said to be. It seems that ginkgo is no exception.

ConsumerLab, an independent testing laboratory in White Plains, New York, analyzes various products for a fee. In recent tests on various brands of ginkgo, they found that only 22 percent met quality standards. Most products contained only one-fifth of the active ingredient claimed on the label. This is a marked drop from the 75 percent that had passing grades in 1999. Only two of the nine brands randomly selected passed the test. These were Maxi Ginkgo Biloba and Nature's Way Ginkgold. A third company that requested and paid for its product to be analyzed, Nutrilite Ginkgo Biloba, also satisfied the standard.

Here's the quandary: As the gingko debate continues among scientists, consumers face the additional possibility that, even if the herb does work, they have no way of knowing whether the brand they use contains enough active ingredient.

THE BOTTOM LINE

Should you be taking ginkgo? If you're healthy, don't waste your money on it. This herb won't do anything for you, even though there is some evidence that it may improve blood flow to various organs of the body, including the brain. Because AD has so few treatment alternatives anyway, I see no harm in someone with AD taking ginkgo even though to date, there is no proof that it has an effect. Remember, however, that this herb is a mild blood thinner, so use it with caution if you're also taking an anticoagulant. Also, discontinue it before having any surgery.

Claims that herbal supplements offer miracle benefits are often not backed up by scientific testing. Even when they are, you still don't know what you're getting when you pick a bottle off a shelf, because it may not contain what the label says it does. ▪

ARTHRITIS

Does Tylenol Really Help Osteoarthritis?

OSTEOARTHRITIS, the degeneration of the body's joints due to wear and tear over the years, is a major cause of disabling pain in older men and women. Although physiotherapy can help, most patients require painkillers. These range from something as simple as aspirin and Tylenol (acetaminophen) to nonsteroidal anti-inflammatory drugs (NSAIDs) to potent narcotics. Always start with the least potent drugs.

Tylenol is generally safe and non–habit-forming, which is why it is available over the counter and usually recommended as the first drug to try for relief of "the aches and pains of minor arthritis," as referred to in the TV commercials. Although the drug is easier on the stomach than many NSAIDs and aspirin, Tylenol overdose is one of the leading causes of poisoning cases that report to emergency rooms in this country. Exceeding the recommended dose can hurt the liver, so be careful if you have a drinking problem or any kind of liver disease.

Despite the widespread use of Tylenol, questions have recently been raised about its effectiveness against the pain of osteoarthritis because osteoarthritic pain is now believed to be caused not only by long-term joint use but also by inflammation. Unlike the NSAIDs and the newer COX-2 inhibitors, such as Celebrex (rofecoxib), Vioxx (valdecoxib), and Bextra (celecoxib), Tylenol does not reduce inflammation. It acts on the nerves that transmit pain.

The manufacturer, however, insists that Tylenol works, and so do millions of patients. Are they right, or is the benefit they describe all in the head?

■ HERE'S WHAT'S NEW

Researchers at the Rush Medical College in Chicago compared the efficacy of Tylenol and anti-inflammatory drugs in 82 men and women with painful osteoarthritis of the knee. One-third of the subjects were given 1,000 milligrams of generic acetaminophen four times a day, another third received 75 milligrams of the NSAID Voltaren (diclofenac) twice daily. The rest took a placebo. Neither the researchers nor the patients knew which groups got which pills.

Using standard measures to determine pain and the stage of the arthritis at the beginning of the study and again after 2 and 12 weeks, researchers assessed the results of each treatment. Guess what? Those taking the NSAID significantly improved, whereas those taking either acetaminophen or placebo did not. What's more, there was *no* difference in the results obtained between the placebo and acetaminophen groups! I can understand a better result from the NSAID than from the Tylenol, but no benefit whatsoever from the Tylenol really surprises me. The researchers concluded that "acetaminophen use in subjects with osteoarthritis of the knee should be reconsidered pending further studies."

■ THE BOTTOM LINE

I don't believe this is the last word on the subject. Tylenol is so popular and so widely used that other studies will certainly test how well it relieves osteoarthritis pain. For now, I recommend that if Tylenol works for you, you should stay with it. If, however, your pain does not respond, don't assume that it's because your arthritis is bad or getting worse. Don't increase the dose of Tylenol and run the risk of toxicity. Switch to an NSAID, taking it, as directed, *after* meals or with milk, to avoid stomach irritation.

A final piece of advice: Don't confuse the painkilling properties of Tylenol with its ability to reduce an elevated temperature. The osteoarthritis study did not address the latter problem. If you're running a fever, Tylenol will reduce it.

WHAT THE DOCTOR ORDERED?

ARNICA FOR PAIN ■ When I was an undergraduate student at McGill University in Montreal, I was passionate about football (watching not playing). My admiration and envy for friends on the team changed to sympathy in the locker room after the game when I saw how bruised and battered they were. Yet, their spirits seemed undiminished as they applied arnica compresses to their aching bodies. (Some also took homeopathic tablets.)

Years later, while in medical school, I was surprised that I was taught nothing about this miracle medication, also called leopard's bane. After graduation and throughout my residency, I never once saw it used in the hospital, where pain of all kinds is treated. Was there some kind of conspiracy by those in evidence-based medicine against all the "wisdom" offered by many "natural" therapies used throughout the ages? These stubborn teachers of mine, and later my colleagues in practice, for some reason insisted on proof of effectiveness before prescribing or recommending any medication, including arnica, whether or not it required a prescription.

In later years, as my immediate relationship to the football field and my contact with its players waned, I forgot about arnica. I treated my pain patients with the gamut of conventional agents ranging from aspirin and Tylenol (acetaminophen) all the way to OxyContin (oxycodone), depending on how much they hurt.

Then, a few years ago, I wrote a book called *Dr. Rosenfeld's Guide to Alternative Medicine*. I based it on a careful review of the scientific literature about, among many other things, arnica. It's still widely used, especially by athletes, just as it was when I was in college some 50 years ago. But I could find no convincing evidence that it really works. In 1998, findings from eight well-controlled trials reported in the *Archives of Surgery* concluded that arnica exerts only a placebo effect despite innumerable testimonials to its effectiveness.

I was at my local health food store the other day to buy some glucosamine and chondroitin for my aching knee when I saw some arnica on a shelf. I asked the owner how well it was selling. "Great," he replied, "as always." I asked him whether his customers preferred the tablets or the topical solutions. "Both," he answered, "but I think the tablets are better."

I decided to review the subject again, this time on the Internet, because I had exhausted all my scientific sources when I wrote my book on alternative medicine. I was amazed to find at site after site, almost all of which were hosted by purveyors of the product or homeopathic practitioners, claims that arnica cures or improves the following conditions, to list just a few: coronary artery disease, a weak immune system, bumped and bruised tissue, arthritis pain, chapped lips, acne, irritated nostrils, fever, dry skin, fluid retention, dry cough (it's apparently an expectorant, too), arteries in spasm, and fatigue (it's also a stimulant). Wow! What a track record for just a single herb! No wonder homeopaths are so keen about it.

I was curious to see what our stick-in-the-mud FDA had to say about arnica. It seems that the government strongly believes that oral preparations of arnica, other than the diluted homeopathic strengths, are unsafe and contain substances that can actually hurt the heart and vascular system, cause violent toxic gastroenteritis, nervous disturbances, intense muscle weakness, contact dermatitis, collapse, and death. So why aren't these toxic oral preparations banned? Because they aren't classified as drugs. Considered "natural supplements," they are not under FDA control. Although the FDA does not question the safety of the topical applications of arnica or the homeopathic oral preparations, it does not endorse their effectiveness either.

HERE'S WHAT'S NEW

The following is for all the arnica enthusiasts who swear by both its oral and topically applied forms. Researchers at the University of Exeter and the Royal Devon and Exeter Hospital in the United Kingdom conducted a rigorous double-blind study of three groups of patients with carpal tunnel syndrome (a painful disorder of the wrist) who took arnica by mouth for 1 week before and 2 weeks after surgery. One group was given high-potency arnica tablets; another group, low-potency tablets; the remaining third, a placebo. Neither the participants nor the doctors treating them knew who was getting what. The patients filled out standard pain-assessment questionnaires throughout the experiment. Their wrists were also photographed at every stage to document the degree of swelling and exact shades of bruising.

After all evidence was in, the researchers concluded that there was "no significant difference" among the groups in terms of bruising, swelling, pain, and the number of painkillers used. There were no toxic effects either.

The researchers recommend that if you hurt for whatever reason, you should use more effective treatment and save money by not buying homeopathic arnica. When asked to explain the large number of anecdotal kudos for this herb, they point out that no two people react to pain in the same way. Those who normally recover quickly anyway and take arnica rave about it to their friends. The nonresponders simply keep mum—and that's how a legend is born and perpetuated.

In all fairness, most homeopaths do not recommend the herb for postoperative pain, so this study should not be taken as a definitive assessment of arnica's use in mild to moderate muscle strain or bruising.

In this study, published in the *Journal of the Royal Society of Medicine*, only oral arnica was used. I'm sorry that they did not evaluate topical arnica. I just can't believe that the entire McGill football team was wrong.

THE BOTTOM LINE

If friends on your college or home football team are applying arnica to their bruised bodies and are happy with it, more power to them. They should stay with it. It can do no harm unless they develop contact dermatitis, and they'll know that soon enough. However, neither you nor they should take arnica by mouth (other than the diluted homeopathic preparations labeled as such) because, as far as the FDA is concerned, it is dangerous.

ASTHMA

Respect the Common Cold

VIRUSES THAT CAUSE THE COMMON COLD (of which there are more than 200) must have an inferiority complex. Even though they make millions of adults and kids miserable at least once a year, no one really worries about them. The flu, a migraine, diarrhea—almost any other common sign or symptom usually warrants a day off, but you're expected to carry on when you have only a "cold." Try telling your boss that you're staying home because you have a cold! Even worse, try telling him or her that you aren't coming to work because your *child* has a cold!

No matter how sick you feel, don't bother taking medication, at least according a recent study in which cough medications and decongestants were found to be of no use whatsoever (see page 70). Oh, and just try asking your doctor for an antibiotic (which, incidentally, most people do and sometimes even succeed in getting). You're sure to receive a lecture about how antibiotics don't work against viruses and why it's important to save them for when you're "really sick."

■ HERE'S WHAT'S NEW

It turns out that the common cold can pack a more powerful punch than we thought—at least for children with asthma. Researchers at the University of Iowa College of Medicine are strongly advising parents of asthmatic children to keep oral steroids handy and to give them to their kids at the first sign of a cold. The scientists have found that doing so greatly reduces the risk of an asthma emergency down the line. Any kind of respiratory infection—everything from "just a cold" to the "real" flu—can trigger serious asthma attacks. Kids younger than age 5 are five times more likely to be hospitalized with the complications of asthma unless they are promptly treated with an oral steroid (the drugs most commonly used for this purpose are prednisone or prednisolone)—and the sooner, the better. That means always keeping some on hand. Such prompt treatment can prevent up to 90 percent of emergency asthma visits to the hospital.

Results from a different but related short-term study also reassure parents not to worry about the complications of oral steroids used briefly from time to time for the treatment of acute respiratory symptoms. Researchers at McGill University Health Center in Montreal found that these medications do not affect bone density or result in any difference in the growth or weight of children who received as many as 11 short courses of such therapy for as long as 1 year.

■ THE BOTTOM LINE

If you have an asthmatic child, ask your doctor about keeping a supply of oral steroids on hand. At the earliest signs of a cold, start treatment for a few days. The sooner you do so, the less likely your child will be to develop a severe asthma attack. Unless you have this medication readily available, symptoms that start after the pharmacies close on Saturday may go untreated until Monday morning, when the drug stores re-open—and that's too long. Note, however, that this recommendation applies only to children with asthma—not all children.

When Asthma Doesn't Respond to Medication

SOME ASTHMATIC KIDS are in and out of emergency rooms with acute respiratory distress because their asthma hasn't responded to maximal doses of any medication. This resistance to conventional treatment has always been interpreted as evidence that their disease is severe.

We have long known that in many adult asthmatics, acid reflux into the esophagus, or gastroesophageal reflux disease (GERD), causes chronic cough and hoarseness independent of their respiratory disease. Indeed their asthma typically improves after the acid reflux is treated.

■ HERE'S WHAT'S NEW

Doctors at the West Jefferson Medical Center in New Orleans theorized that children with persistent moderate asthma who also have GERD might have fewer respiratory symptoms if their acid reflux were treated. They studied 46 asthmatic children, 27 of whom had GERD. They treated most of the latter group with either anti-GERD therapy, such as acid-suppressing drugs (proton pump inhibitors) or surgical correction for the few who needed it.

Here's how this therapy affected their asthma after 12 months: Overall, the asthmatic children treated for GERD needed 50 percent fewer bronchodilators. During the last 6 months of the study, 89 percent took no inhaled steroids. None required leukotriene receptor antagonists (see page 26). By contrast, asthmatic children whose GERD was not treated required the same respiratory medications they had taken all along. Even more interesting, eight of the children who did not have GERD but who chose to receive treatment for it anyway also required less anti-asthma medication.

■ THE BOTTOM LINE

No one really knows why treating GERD reduces symptoms of asthma. But the results of this study, published in *Chest* (the official peer-reviewed journal of the American College of Chest Physicians), strongly suggest that asthmatics who have GERD—and maybe even those who don't have it—should take medication that reduces the amount of acid produced by the stomach. Doing so appears to reduce the severity of their disease and the amount of anti-asthma medication required.

WHAT THE DOCTOR ORDERED?

THE HYGIENE HYPOTHESIS ■ For the past several years, many doctors have wondered why the incidence of asthma and allergies has been rising, especially in developed countries such as the United States. One possible explanation is that, in keeping with our "higher standard of living," we compulsively overprotect our children against relatively harmless infectious organisms and irritants. Keeping bedrooms free from dust, mites, and molds, and scrupulously avoiding contact with other children who have colds and other infections may be the wrong thing to do.

HERE'S WHAT'S NEW

Asthma and allergy researchers at the National Jewish Medical and Research Center in Denver as well as specialists elsewhere believe that our emphasis on cleanliness and hygiene is making us more vulnerable to asthma and allergies. In their opinion, children need some exposure to infectious organisms so that their immune systems can be prepared against more serious attacks later in life. Overprotecting them early on leaves them with no experience in coping with relatively harmless irritants and infectious agents that normally stimulate antibody formation. This lack of protection may result in asthma and allergy years down the line.

The Denver research team found strong evidence to support the hygiene hypothesis with experiments on mice, a group of whom they injected with a bacterium that commonly causes pneumonia. Another group of the mice received a placebo. Two weeks later, both groups of mice were rendered allergic to an egg protein and their respective responses were evaluated. The animals that had been infected with the bacterium had a much milder reaction to the egg protein than did the controls. Their levels of gamma interferon (a synthetic version of a substance that the body produces naturally to help fight infections and tumors) were also higher than in the healthy, nonallergic animals.

Even though mice are not men, these doctors believe that this controlled experiment supports the hypothesis that sparing children a little dust and dirt—or even exposure a bug or two—can leave them more allergic and vulnerable to more serious problems later on.

I discussed this theory with two of my grandchildren, ages 7 and 11, who had just been told to clean up their rooms. They heartily agree with the researchers and now beg to let a little dust accumulate here and there, especially in their own living quarters.

THE BOTTOM LINE

Once a person becomes asthmatic or allergic, it's important to avoid exposure to dust, mites, mold, and infection. However, early in life, small doses of these "contaminants" help the body's immune system develop antibodies when it's challenged later on. Keep your house clean, by all means, but don't overprotect your children. ▪

Newer Treatment Not Always Better

FOR YEARS, most people with mild to moderate asthma took an inhaled corticosteroid to reduce the swelling and inflammation of the nasal and respiratory passages associated with their attacks. Examples include Flonase or Flovent (fluticasone propionate).

More recently, newer drugs called leukotriene receptor antagonists (like Singulair) have gained popularity in the United States and are commonly used in place of inhaled steroids. Leukotrines, like histamines, are substances released when the body is challenged by something to which it is allergic, and that cause the symptoms of allergy. Leukotrine receptor antagonists (LTRAs) are used in the same way as antihistamines to treat these symptoms.

The popularity of LTRAs may be the result of a combination of effective advertising and confusion regarding the safety of inhaled versus oral steroids. Oral steroids can cause serious adverse reactions when taken in large doses for prolonged periods of time; inhaled steroids do not.

Complementary (alternative) medicine devotees believe that homeopathic remedies also improve quality of life for people with mild to moderate asthma and various other disorders. Indeed, such remedies are given to 15 percent of asthmatic children in the United Kingdom. The number in this country is probably less but still substantial. However, most conventional health providers are not convinced of the benefits of homeopathy in asthmatics.

▪ HERE'S WHAT'S NEW

Researchers at McGill University Health Center found the newer nonsteroidal, antileukotrienes less effective than inhaled steroids. Adults with asthma so treated were 60 percent more likely to have flare-ups, night awakenings, and daytime symptoms.

Recently, the University of Exeter's department of complemen-

tary medicine conducted a double-blind study of 93 asthmatic children in southwest England. Homeopathic remedies given by experienced, classically trained homeopaths and continued for 1 year
were found to be no more effective than placebos.

▪ THE BOTTOM LINE

If you have mild to moderate asthma that is well-controlled by an
inhaled corticosteroid that you tolerate well, stay with it. Don't confuse it with the oral steroids. If you do decide to try an an-
tileukotriene such as Singulair and it works, fine. If it doesn't,
however, don't hesitate to go back to the inhaled steroids. They are
safe, and their adverse effects are minimal.

If you've been thinking about homeopathy to help your asthma,
it will leave you breathless. There are better ways to spend your time
and money.

ATTENTION-DEFICIT HYPERACTIVITY DISORDER

New Treatment, New Approach

ATTENTION-DEFICIT HYPERACTIVITY DISORDER (ADHD) is a common behavioral abnormality that starts in childhood, affects 4 to 6 percent of all Americans, and continues throughout life in up to two-thirds of all cases. Kids with ADHD can't focus their attention on anything for long, they're impulsive (if they want something, they have to have it right away), and they can't sit still.

Is ADHD a real disorder or just a variation of normal behavior? According to federal legislation, ADHD is officially a disability, meaning that anyone so diagnosed is entitled to help—in school and at work. Digital imaging studies and positron emission tomography (PET) scans of the brains of people with ADHD have shown that areas that control attention and inhibit impulses are less active and use less sugar for energy than do other parts of the brain. Also, ADHD runs in families: If one family member has ADHD, there is a 25 to 35 percent chance that another will too, compared with only a 4 to 6 percent probability for someone in the general population.

Still, some doctors think that ADHD is overdiagnosed; others deny that it's really a disease. (We used to think that sugar is responsible for hyperactivity, but that's apparently so in only 5 percent of kids). There is also considerable (and occasionally passionate) disagreement about how to treat ADHD. Most observers agree that children with the classic signs of this disorder—fidgeting, squirming, talking a blue streak, blurting out answers to questions that haven't been asked—should have behavioral and cognitive therapy. However, many specialists have serious doubts about what they consider to be an overuse of stimulant medications, such as Ritalin, Dexedrine, and Adderall. Some experts believe that Ritalin is responsible for addiction, that it disrupts growth hormone, and that it may cause physical damage to the brain. For these reasons, the following news is welcome.

■ HERE'S WHAT'S NEW

The FDA has approved a new drug, Strattera (atomoxetine), as a safe, effective treatment for ADHD in patients of all age-groups. It is the first *nonstimulant* medication designated for this purpose. Strattera works by blocking the brain's reabsorption of norepinephrine, a neurotransmitter that moves messages between brain cells and regulates attention, impulsivity, and activity levels. The standard dose is one or two capsules a day, and adverse effects are minimal, typically involving loss of appetite and, rarely, an allergic reaction.

Another interesting study has concluded that children with ADHD respond better to medication and therapy if they also receive biofeedback. When hooked up to a device that measures brain wave activity, these children had better attention spans and behavior ratings, as well as measurable improvement of images of their brain activity, than those who weren't. In some children, this improvement continued for 2 years after completing 40 sessions of biofeed-back. The researchers suggest that biofeedback may be especially helpful for kids who don't tolerate drugs well or who may have trouble stopping their medication because of a family history of addiction.

▪ THE BOTTOM LINE

If your child (or you, for that matter) has been diagnosed with ADHD, is being treated with a stimulant drug, and is not happy with this therapy for whatever reason, you now have a alternative. Ask your doctor about nonstimulant Strattera. Also, consider a course of biofeedback therapy because it appears to enhance the effectiveness of medication.

BAD BREATH

New Strategies for Fresher Breath

BREATH ALWAYS HAS SOME ODOR TO IT—sometimes even a pleasant one. Unfortunately, it also can be offensive. Bad breath (or halitosis) can result from many different causes. Following are the ones we usually think about first:

- Sinus infections, usually with a postnasal drip

- Infected tonsils in children

- Chronic lung disease with mucus in the airways

- Kidney and liver disease caused by odorous waste products that accumulate in the blood and circulate through the body (bad breath ensues when they reach the lungs and are exhaled)

- Infections in the mouth, especially the teeth and gums

- Acidic foods, caffeine, and fish (garlic and onions cause only temporary halitosis)

Halitosis is big business. Pharmacies and health food stores offer a slew of products—special chewing gums, mints, mouthwashes, and sprays—that promise to "freshen" your breath (and allow you to use words that start with the letter *H* in intimate conversations). Few of them work for more than a couple of minutes. In fact, a mouthwash that contains alcohol may make things worse. Brushing your teeth more frequently won't help much either. The only effective way to control bad breath is to eliminate whatever infection may be causing it.

■ HERE'S WHAT'S NEW

Researchers at Baskent University in Turkey have observed that patients with *H. pylori* infection of the stomach frequently have halitosis. (This bacterium is commonly present in the stomach and has been implicated as a possible cause of gastric ulcers, bleeding, and even cancer.) They studied 148 men and women who had *H. pylori* and various gastrointestinal signs and symptoms, such as indigestion, bloating, and burping. About 60 percent of them also had halitosis. After their *H. pylori* was eradicated with the appropriate antibiotic, many of the subjects with halitosis reported that their bad breath had cleared up. So, if your breath is offensive and you have stomach "trouble," ask your doctor to check you for *H. pylori* with a simple blood test or breath analysis. If the results are abnormal and there is no other explanation for the halitosis, have the *H. pylori* treated with an antibiotic. That may not only clean your breath but also help prevent more serious stomach problems later on.

Here's another way to freshen your breath. Researchers at Pace University in New York City and at the University of Illinois have found that a cup of tea can do the trick by fighting oral infection. In the Pace University study, when green tea was added to cultures of the bacteria that cause strep throat and tooth decay, it destroyed almost 100 percent of the organisms. The researchers believe that the tea's polyphenol content acts on the bacteria. They suggest that toothpaste manufacturers add these polyphenols to toothpaste and mouthwash to protect the mouth against infection (and the bad breath that accompanies it).

In the University of Illinois study, researchers exposed three types of mouth bacteria that cause bad breath to black tea and found that the tea reduced their growth by 30 percent. They suggest rinsing your mouth regularly with black tea to reduce plaque formation and halitosis.

■ THE BOTTOM LINE

More and more doctors routinely test patients with upper gastrointestinal symptoms or peptic ulcer disease for *H. pylori* bacteria. If your bad breath persists even after you've eliminated some of its more common causes, have yourself checked for *H. pylori* (especially if you have chronic indigestion or other stomach complaints, too). Treatment of *H. pylori* requires only 10 to 14 days of an antibiotic, several different regimens of which are available.

Being treated for *H. pylori* is the first course of action. Then, get into the habit of drinking tea—green or black. Both types contain polyphenols, which inhibit the bacterial and viral growth responsible for oral infection and bad breath. If you'd rather not drink the tea, just rinse your mouth regularly with it. It happens to be a good mouthwash.

BODY ODOR

Yet Another Use for Botox—
Who Would Have Thought?

MANY YEARS AGO WHEN I WAS A MEDICAL STUDENT, we learned about a condition called botulism. Caused by a toxin from the bacterium *Clostridium botulinum*, this illness can lead to paralysis and even death. You get it by eating contaminated canned foods that have a low acid content, such as asparagus, green beans, beets, and corn (usually canned at home). The clostridium spores can also be present in honey.

There are only about 100 cases of botulism a year in the United States, so it's no surprise that I've never seen a case in all the years I've been practicing medicine. Still, I've always had a healthy respect for this infection. I think of it whenever I see a patient with any of its classic signs or symptoms—double vision, blurred vision, drooping eyelids, slurred speech, difficulty swallowing, a severely dry mouth, and muscle weakness (even though they are more commonly the result of a stroke of some kind).

So imagine my shock a few years ago when I began hearing about all the wonderful things that this deadly poison can do. It has found respectability—even admiration and gratitude—under the commercial name Botox. It turns out that a very, very diluted strength can help erase wrinkles when injected into the skin. Men and women are flocking to their cosmetic gurus for facial Botox treatments. If you know someone who's had the procedure, you'll surely have noticed the bland, expressionless look that often results, reminiscent of the loss of facial expression in patients with Parkinson's disease. I'm not knocking Botox, mind you, because beauty is in the eyes of the beholder.

There is a more tangible upside to Botox than its cosmetic results. It can help relieve migraine headaches by relaxing facial muscles and also can reduce excessive underarm perspiration when injected there.

■ HERE'S WHAT'S NEW

Chalk up another victory to this dreaded toxin. German researchers have discovered that Botox not only reduces underarm perspiration but also virtually eliminates its offensive odors. It isn't clear how it works; it may interfere with skin bacteria or act on the nerves of the sweat glands. Whatever the mechanism, it gets rid of the smell, and that's what counts.

■ THE BOTTOM LINE

If you know that you generate offensive underarm odors (bad enough so that your best friend tells you about it), try a variety of powerful antiperspirants first. If none work and your social life is going down the drain, ask your doctor about Botox treatments.

But remember this: Whether for "beauty" or for treatment of any of the other disorders I've mentioned, this is not a one-shot deal—you need to receive Botox injections every few months for continued results. And it doesn't come cheap!

BREAST CANCER

Minimize Your Risk with Ibuprofen

BREAST CANCER IS THE MOST COMMON MALIGNANCY in women (excluding nonmelanoma skin cancer) and the second leading cause of cancer deaths among them, killing some 40,000 women a year. (Breast cancer will also strike close to 1,300 men this year, 400 of whom will die of it.) In 2004, at least 200,000 new cases of invasive breast cancer will be diagnosed in the United States, along with about 50,000 noninvasive breast cancers confined to the milk ducts. (This type lies dormant for a long time and may never spread, but who wants to chance it? So it is typically removed as soon as it is found.)

Although early detection is the key to successful treatment of breast cancer, its prevention is even more desirable. In that regard, we have been able to identify certain risk factors that increase your chances of developing it. Here are the most important ones.

Age. The danger of developing breast cancer increases as one grows older. There is 1 in 252 chance that a female born today will develop breast cancer between ages 30 and 40; the risk is 1 in 68 between ages 40 and 50, and 1 in 27 between ages 60 and 70. By age 85, her lifetime chance of developing breast cancer is 1 in 8.

Genetics. About 10 percent of breast cancers are hereditary. If your mother, sister, or daughter had breast cancer, you're at twice the risk of developing it too. You can determine your genetic vulnerability by being tested for mutations of the BRCA1 and BRCA2 genes. Mutations of either gene indicate an increased risk of both breast and ovarian cancers.

Previous breast cancer. A previous history of cancer in one breast triples or quadruples your chances of developing cancer in the other.

Hormones. The hormone estrogen, which is produced by the ovaries, is believed to be directly related to the risk of breast cancer. That's why women who've had one or both ovaries removed are less likely to develop this cancer later on in life. And the longer your ovaries have been making estrogen, the greater your risk. Estrogen production drops during pregnancy. So if your estrogen supply has been uninterrupted because you've never had children, you're at higher risk for breast cancer. (That's presumably why nuns are so vulnerable to this malignancy.) Conversely, the more kids you've had and the earlier in life you had them, the lower your risk.

For the same reason, 5 or more years of hormone replacement therapy raises the incidence of breast cancer. Whether taking birth control pills also does is still under debate.

Drugs like Nolvadex (tamoxifen) suppress estrogen production or action and thus reduce the likelihood of breast cancer. Remember, however, that this drug increases the risk of uterine cancer, stroke, and blood clots in the veins, so consider the risk-benefit ratio before deciding whether to take it.

Radiation history. We tend to think of radiation as a treatment against cancer. But radiation also can predispose a person to cancer anywhere in the body, including the breast. If you received radiation during childhood for any reason (Hodgkin's disease, thyroid problems, even acne), you may be more vulnerable to breast cancer. It's also a good reason to think twice about having routine chest x-rays, especially in children.

Unfortunately, you can't do much about such risk factors as your age, genetics, or family history. But you do have control over some others. For example, reconsider hormone replacement therapy. Fewer women take it these days, not only because it raises the risk of cancer but also because earlier assessments of its benefits have not been substantiated (see page 181). As far as the Pill is concerned, the possibility of increased danger of breast cancer arising from its use is so small that it should not affect your decision to take it.

Various lifestyle modifications also can reduce your risk. For example, exercising regularly may reduce your hormone levels. Breastfeeding your children is also helpful. Although drinking alcohol raises the risk somewhat, the benefits of moderate alcohol intake probably outweigh the breast cancer risk. Cigarette smoking is bad for you for other reasons, and a study published in April 2001 found that smoking significantly increases the risk of breast cancer in women with a strong family history of breast and ovarian cancers.

Your diet may be important on two accounts. First, gaining weight increases your risk, especially after menopause. Second, populations that eat a high-fat diet have a higher incidence of breast cancer. However, I am not aware of any studies confirming that a low-fat diet reduces the risk.

As a last resort, if you have a host of significant risk factors—such as the presence of mutated BRCA1 and BRCA2 genes; a strong family history of breast cancer, ovarian cancer, or both; or recurrent lumps requiring frequent biopsies—you may want to consider having your breasts removed. Doing so appears to reduce the risk of breast cancer by 90 percent. (I'm amazed at how effectively sophisticated breast reconstruction techniques restore the appearance of the chest in such patients.)

■ HERE'S WHAT'S NEW

Many of the above observations are relatively recent. However, you should know about an important new one. An Ohio State University study of 80,000 postmenopausal women ages 50 to 79 revealed that those who took a single 200-milligram tablet of ibuprofen (the most popular brand names are Motrin and Advil) two or more times a week for at least 10 years reduced their risk of breast cancer by 49 percent. Aspirin worked too, but not as effectively. A single 325-milligram tablet taken the same way as the ibuprofen reduced the incidence of breast cancer in these women by 22 percent. This was true even for women with strong family histories and other risk factors. Tylenol (acetaminophen), a painkiller but not an anti-inflammatory, had no effect on the incidence of breast cancer.

The lead researcher believes that anti-inflammatory drugs probably work against other cancers as well. In fact, other studies have shown that anti-inflammatories help prevent cancers of the colon by 20 to 30 percent, and may also protect against heart attacks and Alzheimer's disease.

The researchers don't entirely understand the protective effect of anti-inflammatories. They suspect the drugs may prevent cancer by blocking harmful gene mutations and the spread of cancer cells, and may also speed the death of malignant cells.

■ THE BOTTOM LINE

There are some risk factors for breast cancer about which you can do little or nothing. Others, such as lifestyle and diet, are under your control. The latest finding indicates that an over-the-counter painkiller, such as the anti-inflammatory drug ibuprofen, taken only twice a week over a 10-year period can reduce the incidence of this malignancy by almost half, as can a single aspirin tablet, albeit somewhat less effectively. If there is no reason for you not to take these medications on a regular basis (bleeding disorders, gastrointestinal problems, allergic reaction to the drugs, and anticoagulant therapy are contraindicated), ask your doctor about the pros and cons of doing so—especially if you are at high risk for breast cancer.

Pregnancy Loss Not a Risk Factor

FOR MANY YEARS a National Cancer Institute (NCI) fact sheet stated that there is "no causal association between abortion and breast cancer." Then, toward the end of 2002, it revised that conclusion to read that any linkage between induced abortions and breast cancer was "inconclusive." Now, in an even newer version of the fact sheet, the NCI states that abortion, induced or spontaneous (the latter including miscarriage), is *not* associated with any increase in breast cancer risk.

Why was the possibility of a link between pregnancy loss and breast cancer ever raised in the first place? It was all highly theoretical. Here's how the logic went: There appears to be an association between exposure to estrogen and the incidence of breast cancer. As mentioned earlier, the longer a woman has high concentrations of estrogen circulating through her body, the greater her risk of breast cancer. During pregnancy, those hormone levels fall—and that's good as far as breast cancer is concerned. Conversely, when the pregnancy is terminated for any reason, there is more estrogen again. So, at least theoretically, an interrupted pregnancy could increase the risk of breast cancer later in life.

▪ HERE'S WHAT'S NEW

Four substantial studies and a review of several earlier ones were evaluated at an NCI workshop in early 2003 by a specially appointed scientific panel. Despite the theoretical speculation I described above, these experts concluded that there is no proof that abortion increases the risk of breast cancer. One study involving 1.5 million Danish women concluded that those who'd had induced abortions were not at increased risk of breast cancer. Earlier reports that suggested otherwise were determined to be flawed.

Absolving abortion of this stigma does not weaken the link between estrogen and breast cancer. This same panel also concluded that the more babies a woman has, and the younger she is when her first full-term baby is born, the less likely she is to develop breast cancer. Women who have never given birth have about the same risk of breast cancer as those who delivered their firstborns at age 30.

▪ THE BOTTOM LINE

The number of terminated pregnancies a woman has had—whether induced or natural—has no bearing whatsoever on her risk of developing breast cancer later on. This fear should not prey on her mind. Regardless of her obstetric history, every woman should be screened for breast cancer starting at age 40. How often to do so (and whether to be screened *before* age 40) depends on the presence of other risk factors.

WHAT THE DOCTOR ORDERED?

THE MAMMOGRAM DEBATE ▪ For years, routine mammography has been a way of life for most American women. That's because (1) breast cancer is a leading cause of death among them, (2) mammography detects many small cancers up to 2 years earlier than manual breast examinations do, and (3) early diagnosis increases the chance of a cure. So it would seem indisputable that vulnerable females (typically those age 40 and older) should have an annual mammogram. Right? Not necessarily, according to some observers.

Who dares challenge this advice? Lots of people. First, there are the "cost effectiveness" types, forever trying to determine how many lives mammography must save in order to make it "worthwhile." Then there are the statisticians, analyzing numbers to determine how "reliable" the mammogram is in diagnosing breast cancer and whether screening really makes any difference to overall survival. Then there are "experts" who question whether the mammogram is, in fact, the best way to diagnose breast cancer—and whether women should use another technique either instead of or in addition to it. Finally, some oncologists claim that early detection makes no difference in the long run for many breast cancers, and that there is plenty of time to treat tumors after they are large enough to be felt.

Each reservation about mammography has some validity. However, are they sufficiently relevant to preclude having an annual mammogram? It depends. Whether or not mammograms save enough lives to justify the expenditure depends on one's personal experience. What do you think would be the opinion of someone in whom such a cancer was picked up in a mammogram, treated in time, and cured?

Given these differences of opinion, many women are confused about having regular mammograms. However, most practicing doctors like me have stuck to their guns and continued to advise their patients to be routinely screened.

Over the years, despite the occasional negative conclusion, most researchers have continued to recommend routine mammography. Seven landmark studies in the 1970s and 1980s found that mammography saves lives. Then, in 2000, came a bombshell. Researchers in Denmark reanalyzed these data and determined that most of them were flawed. When they put all the evidence together, these scientists concluded that the annual mammogram did not, in fact, result in any significant reduction in the death rate from breast cancer. Mammography's detractors had a field day; its proponents were put on the defensive. And that's where the matter stood—until now.

HERE'S WHAT'S NEW

The largest and most credible study ever done to evaluate the impact of routine mammography on survival has concluded that routine mammograms do significantly reduce deaths from breast cancer. Scientists in the United States, Sweden, Britain, and Taiwan compared the number of deaths from breast cancer diagnosed in the 20 years before mammogram screening became available with the number in the 20 years after its introduction. The research was based on the histories and treatment of 210,000 Swedish women ages 20 to 69. The researchers found that death from breast cancer dropped 44 percent in women who had routine mammography. Among those who refused mammograms during this time period there was only a 16 percent reduction in death from this disease (presumably the decrease was due to better treatment of the malignancy).

Researchers at New York's Memorial Sloan-Kettering Cancer Center have found that magnetic resonance imaging (MRI) can detect small breast cancers missed by a mammogram. They recommend that women at high risk undergo *both* types of screening. (High-risk women are defined as those who have previously been treated for breast cancer, have a close relative such as a mother or sister with the disease, have tested positive for *mutations* in the BRCA1 or BRCA2 genes, or have benign breast lumps that could later cause cancer.)

Shortly after the appearance of the Denmark study, the American Cancer Society (ACS) issued its own mammogram guidelines in A *Cancer Journal for Clinicians* (Vol.53, No.3), making no major changes to the previous, 1997 recommendations. It also recommends breast ultrasound, MRI, or both for those at special risk for breast cancer. This organization emphasizes that between ages 20 and 39, women should make sure their doctor performs a manual breast examination at least every 3 years. The ACS continues to endorse annual mammography between ages 40 and 69, except for women who have other serious health problems or a short life expectancy. The problem with mammograms in the 40-to-49 age group is the relatively high number of false-positives, especially in patients with dense breasts.

What about mammography after age 69? I still recommend it to my own patients, but some debate exists among most doctors. Given the shortened life expectancy and higher risk of death from causes other than breast cancer, many doctors conclude that mammography after age 69 is not worthwhile. Some research suggests that bone mineral density can be used to predict the usefulness of mammograms for older women. Because high bone mineral density reflects higher estrogen levels throughout life, it is a good predictor of increased breast cancer risk. When researchers assessed the benefits of screening women age 70 and up, they found that mammograms in those with high bone mineral density would prevent 9.4 cancer deaths in every 10,000 women. Screening women with low bone mineral density would prevent only 1.4 additional deaths per 10,000 women. I present the facts to women in my practice and let them decide whether to continue mammography in their seventies.

The American Cancer Society is much less adamant than it used to be about breast self-examination (BSE). However, I continue to make sure my patients know how to examine their breasts and encouraging them to do so regularly. Over the years, a few of them have detected tumors in the interval between their regularly scheduled mammograms or office visits.

THE BOTTOM LINE

Routine mammograms are important, especially for women between ages 50 and 69. In my own practice, I recommend one every 3 years to all female patients, starting at age 40 and annually thereafter. However, it's important to have a mammogram every year if you're at high risk or have a benign breast tumor.

Women whose breasts are dense should have a sonogram as well as a mammogram to clarify the significance of "suspicious" lumps. The latest research indicates that MRIs are especially useful in high-risk women and reduce the chance of missing a small cancer. It may be wise to have both a mammogram and an MRI if you're at high risk. Given the high cost of MRIs, discuss with your doctor whether just a sonogram (which is much less expensive) without the MRI might provide the answer.

With regard to breast self-examinations, the ACS says it originally recommended them before mammograms were widely available. Some specialists believe that women actually detect breast tumors themselves accidentally—while bathing or dressing—and not during deliberate examination. So rather than have women feel guilty about not examining their own breasts, the ACS says, in effect, "We'll forgive you if you promise to follow the mammogram schedule we recommend." My advice? Do BSEs anyway, but don't be consumed by guilt if you miss them once in a while.

CERVICAL CANCER

What's the Optimal Screening Interval?

A PAP TEST is the most reliable way to detect the early stages of cervical cancer, a malignancy that strikes some 12,000 American women and causes about 4,100 deaths every year, according to the American Cancer Society. The test involves inserting a sterile metal or plastic instrument called a speculum into the vagina to separate the vaginal walls and expose the cervix. A "smear" of cells is obtained from the cervix with a tiny brush or a small spatula and then examined for abnormalities.

For years, the American Cancer Society (ACS) recommended that women get a Pap test every year. To ensure cost-effectiveness, lawmakers and insurance companies continually scrutinize the need for annual screening in healthy women and what intervals are optimal. Because of the low risk of developing cervical cancer, policymakers have been considering the safety of extending that interval to every 2 to 3 years.

■ HERE'S WHAT'S NEW

The ACS and the U.S. Preventive Services Task Force (USPSTF) both have issued a new set of guidelines for cervical cancer screening. They agree that it should begin on an annual basis about 3 years after the onset of sexual activity or at age 21, whichever comes first. (Previous guidelines recommended starting screening at age 18.) At age 30, women who have had three consecutive normal Pap tests may wait 2 to 3 years to have the next one. They made this new recommendation because cervical cancer grows slowly and can still be cured even if it is not detected immediately. Also, more frequent screening, in addition to inducing anxiety, can result in unnecessary biopsies and other procedures.

The new guidelines also suggest that the Pap test may be discontinued at age 65 (it used to be age 70) in women who have not had an abnormal Pap test result any time during the preceding 10 years. However, any woman with HIV or a history of cervical cancer should continue to be tested.

The guidelines for women younger than 65 are supported by a large study of women age 30 to 64 in which testing every three years resulted in an average excess risk of cervical cancer in only three cases in 100,000. These findings were reported in the October 16, 2003 issue of *The New England Journal of Medicine*.

However, researchers at Kaiser Permanente health maintenance organization reviewed the history of 1,416 of their patients, 482 of whom had cervical cancer, and concluded that the risk of missing an early diagnosis of cervical cancer doubles if a woman is screened at 2-to-3-year intervals, instead of once a year.

■ THE BOTTOM LINE

I suggest a compromise. If you're not at special risk, extend the screening interval to three years. But stay with annual testing if you have had questionable findings in the past, or have any problem that compromises your immune system and makes you more vulnerable to cancer.

There's Something Better Than Just a Pap Test

FEW OF MY FEMALE PATIENTS know what the "Pap" in Pap test stands for. But I was surprised when some of my medical students didn't know either. Pap is neither an instrument nor a chemical. It's an abbreviation for the tongue-twisting name George Papanicolaou. He was the doctor who devised the test. My students' lack of awareness is especially surprising not only because the Pap test is one of the most important techniques used in medicine but also because Dr. Papanicolaou did his work at *their* medical school, Weill Cornell Medical College. More than that, his bust sits in the entrance hall through which they pass several times a day! (I try to teach them to be more observant doctors than they are students.)

The Pap test remains the best way to detect the earliest precancerous cell changes in the cervix. Until recently, the only way to be sure of the result was to repeat the test every few months to see whether these suspicious cells cleared up or began to look more like cancer. "Cell abnormalities" reported in a Pap test generate ongoing anxiety, especially when follow-up tests or treatments are recommended for months or even years. The emotional trauma during these intervals is real.

Not every "abnormal" looking cell is destined to become malignant. In a study of almost 350,000 women who underwent routine

Pap testing, British researchers found that when the results warranted further follow-up, 80 percent never developed cancer! These numbers should reassure women that "cell abnormalities" are not a death sentence.

Identifying a woman's previous infection with the human papillomavirus (HPV) also can reduce the need for repeated testing. Close to 100 strains of HPV exist, and they cause various problems, including warts (benign noncancerous tumors) in the genital area and elsewhere. Roughly 30 of the strains are spread through sexual contact and infect an estimated 20 percent of sexually active women in the United States. Some 50 to 75 percent of sexually active adults will have been infected at some point in their lives.

Although HPV infection commonly does not result in longterm health problems, some infected women do go on to develop cervical cancer. Indeed, most patients with cervical cancer test positive for HPV antibodies. This means that if you have a "suspicious" Pap test result but test negative for HPV, you're at little risk for cervical cancer. You should still have a follow-up exam, but less frequently and with much less anxiety. The obvious conclusion is that there is much to be said (other than the cost) for getting an HPV test at the same time that you have your Pap smear.

■ HERE'S WHAT'S NEW

The FDA has approved a new screening method for cervical cancer that does just that. It combines a Pap test with a test that can detect the DNA of the 13 strains of HPV linked with 99 percent of cervical cancers. This technique, called the DNA-withPap and developed by the Digene Corporation, has been shown to be 97.8 percent accurate. By comparison, the Pap test alone is only 70 to 80 percent sensitive in detecting cervical cancer; other HPV testing is 85 to 95 percent reliable. When you combine the two, as the DNAwithPap does, the accuracy is close to 100 percent. A negative DNAwithPap result is a virtual guarantee that you do not have cervical cancer and, what's more, that you're unlikely to develop it (unless, of course, you become infected with HPV at a later date). Preliminary guidelines from the ACS state that a woman who has a negative DNAwithPap result may wait 3 years before having another test. I agree with that recommendation.

In other relevant news about cervical cancer, researchers at the National Cancer Institute believe that long-term use of birth control pills increases the risk of cervical cancer in women who have HPV. Such women should have both a Pap test and an HPV test, or the recently approved DNAwithPap.

■ THE BOTTOM LINE

You may continue to have regular Pap tests as recommended, but for peace of mind, I suggest the new DNAwithPap test that also looks for evidence of the dangerous HPV infection. It's almost 98 percent accurate. Although it costs between $50 and $60 and some insurers won't pay for it, it needs to be done only every 3 years, and you can skip the annual Pap test.

New Hope for Cervical Cancer Survivors Who Want a Family

IF A ROUTINE PAP TEST reveals definite evidence of cervical cancer, and you've had these screens regularly, chances are the disease is at Stage 1 and early enough to cure. You can be optimistic because the data show that over 50 percent of the 12,000 such cancers diagnosed every year in this country are Stage 1, 92 percent of which can be cured.

The best treatment for such a malignancy is removal of the cancer—lock, stock, and barrel. In the past, that almost always meant removing not only the cancerous cervix but the entire uterus as well—in short, a hysterectomy. The problem is, a hysterectomy means no more babies, which obviously is devastating to a woman of childbearing age who has not yet started or completed her family.

An alternative to the hysterectomy is the radical trachelectomy, which preserves a portion of healthy cervix, along with an opening large enough to allow normal menstrual flow. The uterus is left intact. The cervical stump can support the weight of a growing fetus that will be delivered by Cesarean section. However, this more limited operation is generally only offered to women with the early stages of cervical cancer.

■ HERE'S WHAT'S NEW

Our medical culture has focused too long on the radical hysterectomy and radiation as the treatment of choice for cervical cancer in even its early stages. The radical trachelectomy is effective against cancer and it permits women of childbearing age to conceive and deliver healthy babies by Cesarean section. It's important for this message to reach women with early cervical cancer who want to have or continue to bear children.

Doctors at the Albert Einstein College of Medicine in New York City reported to the Annual Clinical Meeting of the American College of Obstetricians and Gynecologists their experience with 32 women with early cervical cancer. All of the patients who underwent the procedure that left the uterus behind had normal periods within the next 3 months, and two of them subsequently delivered normal babies. None had evidence of recurrence of the cancer.

■ THE BOTTOM LINE

If you are of childbearing age and want to have a child but have been diagnosed with Stage 1 cervical cancer, ask your gynecologist whether you are a candidate for a radical trachelectomy, rather than the traditional hysterectomy. Women in whom only the cancer is removed, leaving a portion of cervix behind, can remain fertile. After a 2-year wait, they can become pregnant and have the child by Cesarean section.

CHILDBIRTH COMPLICATIONS

Deliver a Healthy Infant

As MANY AS 25 PERCENT of pregnant women harbor a bacterium known as Group B streptococcus (GBS). Because it may produce no symptoms other than occasional mild urinary complaints, the infection sometimes goes undiagnosed and untreated. (Don't confuse Group B with Group A streptococcus, which typically causes a bad sore throat.)

Although GBS is usually innocuous for the mother, it can be dangerous to an infant who contracts it while passing through the birth canal. In fact, GBS is the most common life-threatening infection of newborns in the United States and a leading cause of their death. Every year, in this country alone, GBS affects more than 1,600 babies at birth. One in 20 of them dies, and those who survive may be left with chronic problems such as poor hearing or vision, learning disabilities, or other neurological disorders.

■ HERE'S WHAT'S NEW

The American College of Obstetricians and Gynecologists now recommends that all pregnant women be screened routinely for GBS with vaginal and rectal swabs between the 35th and 37th weeks of pregnancy. The FDA recently has approved a new, faster test that identifies the infection in an hour. (It used to take up to 2 days to receive test results.) This earlier result will protect the infants of women who, if found to be infected, can then be given intravenous doses of the appropriate antibiotic during labor and before delivery in time to prevent the transmission of GBS to the infant.

■ THE BOTTOM LINE

If you're pregnant, regardless of whether you have symptoms of genitourinary infection, you should be screened in the weeks before your delivery to make sure you are not harboring Group B streptococcus. Most doctors with whom I've spoken do this testing, but ask yours anyway just to be sure. Unfortunately, a few infants become infected despite this therapy, so ask your pediatrician about the warning signs and symptoms of GBS infection (such as pneumonia and meningitis) in the first days of life.

Wait! Prevent Premature Delivery

PRETERM DELIVERY (when the baby is born before the 37th week of pregnancy) is the most important problem facing obstetricians and pregnant women today. Throughout the world, more than 13 million babies are born prematurely every year, and the incidence is rising. In the United States, one out of eight babies is born too soon.

The many consequences of premature delivery range from death of the newborn (especially those born before 30 weeks) to disabilities later in life such as learning delays, cerebral palsy, blindness, and deafness. Even babies born only 2 to 4 weeks before their due dates can experience significant delays in their development, something every woman considering Cesarean section for nonmedical reasons should bear in mind. Women should let nature takes its course unless there is some compelling medical reason to have a preterm Cesarean.

Women at greatest risk for premature labor (1) have a history of previous premature births; (2) are pregnant with twins, triplets, or more; (3) have a less than 6-month gap between pregnancies; or (4) are troubled by chronic uterine or vaginal infections. Other known risk factors that should be controlled include:

- Nutritional deficiencies and consumption of junk food during pregnancy
- Use of alcohol, tobacco, and illicit drugs
- High blood pressure
- Chronic gum disease

Unfortunately, the uterus sometimes unpredictably begins contracting before it should, and the baby is born too soon. Doctors don't always know why this happens, and most of the drugs given to prevent premature labor don't really work. When they do, it's only for a day or two. Bed rest, the old standby, is also usually ineffective.

■ HERE'S WHAT'S NEW

Researchers in Denmark have come up with a fascinating and important observation regarding premature births. They analyzed the obstetrical history of more than 8,000 pregnant women, asking each one how much fish they regularly ate during pregnancy. They found that the more fish eaten, the lower the risk of premature birth—7 percent among those who consumed no fish at all, but only 2 percent in women who ate it once a week!

What is it about fish that offers this protection? It's docosahexa-noic acid (DHA), one of the omega-3 fatty acids present in oily fish such as mackerel, herring, trout, salmon, and sardines. DHA sup-presses the formation of prostaglandins, chemicals that cause the pregnant uterus to contract and are the basis of medications used to stimulate the onset of labor.

Scientists at Wake Forest University in Winston-Salem, North Carolina and 19 other research centers have come up with another important finding of their own. They studied a group of women who had previously delivered at least one baby before 37 weeks. Starting at between 16 and 20 weeks into pregnancy and until the 36th week, the women received either a placebo or weekly injections of the drug 17-alpha-hydroxyprogesterone caproate (17P), a synthetic form of the hormone progesterone. Progesterone levels in the blood nor-mally begin to rise early in pregnancy and continue to do so throughout its course. This hormone makes the uterus less able to contract and relaxes its smooth muscle. At the same time, it builds up the uterine lining and placenta to provide nutrition for the em-bryo and also stimulates the breast glands in preparation for breast-feeding.

The results of this study were very impressive. Women treated with 17P were 42 percent less likely to deliver before 32 weeks and had 34 percent fewer deliveries before 37 weeks than those on placebo. What's more, the incidence of complications among the newborns was also less in the women who had received the drug. The FDA currently approves 17P only for the treatment of infer-tility, not for preventing premature births. If further studies docu-ment these findings, I'm sure that will change.

A pregnant woman's dental health is also an important predictor for full-term delivery. When researchers at the University of Al-abama treated gum infections in 366 pregnant women before their

35th week by scaling and root planing (but not antibiotics), there was an 84 percent reduction of premature births.

■ THE BOTTOM LINE

If you have a history of giving birth prematurely or are vulnerable to doing so because of the risk factors listed above, you should be especially sure you're receiving attentive prenatal care. See your obstetrician regularly, get lots of rest, eat a well-balanced diet, and take all the prenatal vitamins that have been prescribed. Also have your dentist check your mouth for evidence of gum disease. It's not always apparent, and I don't know any obstetricians who check the teeth. Cleaning the teeth and correcting periodontal disease can significantly reduce your risk of going into premature labor. In addition, eat one serving of fish every week or take omega-3 fatty acids in capsule form. Avoid tuna, mackerel, tilefish, swordfish, and shark because of their high mercury content (although canned fish is safe). Ask your doctor whether the FDA has already approved weekly 17P injections between the 16th and 20th weeks of pregnancy for women at high risk for premature labor.

COLD AND FLU

Echinacea—Is It All It's Cracked Up to Be?

THOUSANDS OF CONSUMERS around the world believe that echinacea mobilizes infection-fighting white blood cells in the body and strengthens immune defenses, and therefore helps prevent the common cold and relieve its symptoms. Sales of echinacea account for 10 percent of the billions of dollars spent on herbal supplements in this country. We even keep echinacea in our home medicine cabinet, even though I am not convinced that it really works. But my wife is, so who am I to argue?

■ HERE'S WHAT'S NEW

Two research reports on echinacea about 3 months apart cast doubt on its effectiveness. Let me tell you about them so you can decide for yourself whether this herb is worth taking.

In the first study, reported in the *Annals of Internal Medicine*, doctors at the University of Wisconsin evaluated the effect of echinacea on 148 students who came down with the common cold. In this controlled study, half the students received the herb and the rest were given a placebo. Neither the doctors nor the patients knew who was receiving what. When the results were analyzed, there was no real difference between the treated and placebo groups in terms of the severity of the cold and its duration. In fact, cold symptoms actually lasted a little longer in those receiving the herb. Proponents of echinacea say that these results don't mean much because the researchers used only one type of echinacea (*Echinacea angustifolia*) and their findings may not necessarily apply to other types.

The second paper raises even more doubts as to the wisdom of spending your hard-earned money on echinacea. It looked into the manufacturing process of this herb, given the fact that the FDA doesn't routinely monitor supplements, as it does prescription drugs. Doctors at Presbyterian St. Luke's Hospital in Denver analyzed the contents of echinacea-labeled products sold in retail stores in the Denver area. Among the 59 preparations sampled (21 of which claimed to be standardized, meaning that there is no variation from bottle to bottle), 52 percent contained the ingredients as labeled. A full 10 percent contained no echinacea at all! What's more, among those claiming to be standardized, only 43 percent actually were. All in all, a rather poor showing.

■ THE BOTTOM LINE

If you take echinacea to treat (or prevent) your common cold and you think it works for you, by all means continue to use it, especially if it agrees with you. So what if the benefit you perceive is all in your head? You feel better, don't you? But if you've never been convinced that the herb works for you, yet you continue to spend money on it because everyone (including your wife) tells you it works, use this as the justification for trying something else, such as chicken soup.

Here's an afterthought suggested by my echinacea-hooked wife. She asks, "What if the echinacea preparation that was tested in this study and found to be ineffective was among the 10 percent that didn't contain the active ingredient? In that case, concluding that echinacea doesn't work isn't really justified, is it?" That's a far-fetched possibility, but who ever would have thought of it—other than my wife?

Flu Treatments—New and Old

HERE ARE TWO BASIC FACTS you need to know about the flu virus: (1) Almost everybody should get the flu vaccine. (2) The flu is not caused by a bacterium, so antibiotics won't make you better.

Years ago the flu vaccine was recommended only for the elderly and the chronically sick. However, most doctors now feel that everyone should be protected against its ravages, even if it is not life-threatening to them.

Unfortunately, recent observations indicate that, although older people should be vaccinated against the flu, the vaccine may not protect them as effectively as it does younger people. If you are a senior citizen and were vaccinated, don't dismiss the possibility of flu if you develop its typical signs and symptoms. See your doctor and get treated as early as possible because flu is a major killer of the elderly.

Flu treatment has always consisted basically of reducing the severity of its signs and symptoms—fever, cough, aches, and pains. We take Tylenol (acetaminophen) or Advil (ibuprofen), cough suppressants, and lots of fluids. And don't forget bed rest.

Several anti-flu medications, aimed both at prevention and treatment, were introduced a few years ago. The older ones are Symmetrol (amantadine) and its newer, preferred derivative Flumadine (rimantadine). These pills typically are taken at the earliest onset of symptoms.

Also, if for some reason you can't or won't have the vaccine and have been exposed to the flu, the amantadine family of drugs helps reduce your risk of becoming infected. (They only work against type A flu, not type B.)

Newer medications actually attack the flu virus itself and prevent it from reproducing. One medication, Relenza (zanamivir), is inhaled orally; the other, Tamiflu (oseltamivir), comes in pill form. Both shorten the duration of the infection and reduce the severity of its symptoms. Tamiflu also is approved for preventing flu types A and B in those ages 13 or older.

■ HERE'S WHAT'S NEW

Elderberry has been used for centuries to treat everything from respiratory tract infections to gastrointestinal symptoms to depression. In fact, it has been called the "medicine chest of the common people."

Now comes word from some credible scientists that elderberry really does work against the flu. Researchers at the University of Oslo School of Medicine in Norway have found that an extract from the black elderberry reduces the symptoms and duration of flu types A and B. Flu patients given this herbal extract recovered in about 3 days as compared to 7 days in those taking a placebo. Apparently, an ingredient in elderberry attacks the flu virus and prevents it from attaching to the body's cells and making us sick.

The specific preparation used in this study was developed by an Israeli virologist and is marketed as Sambucol. It may not yet be available in this form in the United States, but ask your health food store if they sell other elderberry preparations. It may be worth trying (along with the conventional medications) if you come down with the flu.

■ THE BOTTOM LINE

Although several effective medications minimize the severity and duration of the flu, there is no cure. You may want to consider taking black elderberry extract, which has recently been shown to be an effective palliative for this infection as soon as the diagnosis is confirmed. But use it along with the proven antiviral agents now available for this infection.

More Flu Shots, Less Death

IT ALWAYS AMAZES ME that so many of my patients resist receiving their annual flu shots. These are the same people who clamor for MRIs, CT scans, colonoscopies, and other time-consuming, expensive, unpleasant procedures, yet balk at getting a little jab in the arm once a year. (Don't get me wrong, these other tests are important, especially the colonoscopy, but it's often easier to "sell" them than it is a flu shot.)

Some of their reasons for rejection are:

A. "I had one last year."

B. "No, sir, never again. I got the flu after the last shot."

C. "Look, doc, I never get the flu."

D. "I'll take it only if I get the flu."

E. "I can't take it because I am allergic to eggs and chicken."

Here's how I respond to each of these excuses.

A. Unlike other vaccinations, such as the one against pneumonia, which lasts for years and usually need not be taken again after age 65, a new formulation of flu vaccine is made annually because the specific flu virus changes from year to year. Last year's supply won't protect you.

B. The flu vaccine contains the dead virus. It cannot cause the flu. If you come down with the infection after you were vaccinated, it's because you were already harboring the bug, and it takes about 2 weeks for the vaccine to work.

C. Everybody is vulnerable to the flu. If you have never had it, it's probably only a matter of time until you do—unless you get the shot.

D. Once you come down with the symptoms, it's too late for the vaccine to work (although now some effective antiviral drugs can reduce the duration of the illness and the severity of its symptoms).

E. Having an allergy to eggs or chicken is the only valid reason not to have the shot.

Every year, more than 100,000 people are hospitalized because of the flu, and 36,000 of them die. Most have not been vaccinated and are older than age 65. The vaccine protects 70 to 90 percent of healthy adults against the flu and prevents it from developing into pneumonia in 50 to 60 percent of the elderly and those with compromised immune systems.

■ HERE'S WHAT'S NEW

The Veterans Affairs Medical Center in Minneapolis, Minnesota, compiled data from 280,000 men and women 65 years and older during flu season in 1998, 1999, and 2000. Those who received a flu shot not only had a 29 to 32 percent lower incidence of pneumonia and flu but also were 19 percent less likely to be hospitalized for heart disease and had 16 to 23 percent fewer hospital admissions for stroke. Overall, a flu shot reduced the risk of dying of any cause by 48 to 50 percent. I wonder if these impressive figures will have any impact on all the naysayers in my practice.

Here's more good news. If you're between ages 5 and 49, you can now be vaccinated with a nasal spray, recently approved by the FDA. No more needles!

Now for some bad news. It seems that the flu vaccine is not quite as effective as we used to think, especially for the elderly. Men and women older than age 80 are many more times likely to develop influenza even after being vaccinated than those 15 to 20 years younger. That's probably because their immune systems are unable to respond to the vaccine and so don't produce enough antibodies to ward off the infection. The practical implications of this observation are that if you are older and were given the vaccine but develop what appears to be the flu, see your doctor about it. Don't assume that it's only a cold simply because you were vaccinated.

■ THE BOTTOM LINE

The flu vaccine remains the number one safeguard against the flu. Young or old, healthy or sick, get vaccinated—but not if you're allergic to eggs or chicken. And if you're between ages 5 and 49, you can have the vaccine as a nasal spray.

No Aspirin for Kids under Age 16

FOR YEARS, doctors in the United States have been warning parents not to give their children aspirin. The reason is a rare disorder called Reye's syndrome, which for some unknown reason can develop in children (and occasionally in adults) who have taken aspirin to relieve symptoms of a recent viral infection, such as the flu, the common cold, or chickenpox. Although Reye's syndrome occurs only in one in a million cases, when it does strike, it can be fatal. It attacks the brain and liver, and unless it is diagnosed early on, it causes death within a few days. There is no cure for Reye's. Treatment typically involves reducing the elevated pressure the disease causes in the brain.

■ HERE'S WHAT'S NEW

Since 1986, the United Kingdom has reduced the incidence of Reye's by banning the use of aspirin for anyone younger than age 12.

The U.K.'s Medicines Control Agency has now expanded the limit to age 16 because of the Reye's-related death of a 13-year-old who is thought to have taken aspirin.

■ THE BOTTOM LINE

Do not give aspirin to any child younger than age 16. Use Tylenol (acetaminophen) instead.

WHAT THE DOCTOR ORDERED?

SHOULD YOU BOTHER TAKING COUGH MEDICINE? ■ The two medications most people ask for when they have a cold or the flu are antibiotics and cough medicine. Doctors now know better than to give you antibiotics at the drop of a hat like they once did. That's because most upper-respiratory infections are due to a virus against which antibiotics are useless. Taking them only increases your likelihood of developing antibiotic resistance, and then when you really need them in the future, they may not work.

Cough medicines are another matter. They usually contain two kinds of ingredients, one to loosen respiratory congestion (an expectorant) and the other to suppress the cough. Surely there isn't any harm in this—or is there?

HERE'S WHAT'S NEW

Representatives of the American College of Physicians–American Society of Internal Medicine, a group that represents more than 100,000 doctors, have concluded that cough syrups are usually a waste of money. There's apparently little or no evidence that the expectorants they contain provide any benefit for upper- or lower-respiratory tract infections (despite the manufacturers' insistence to the contrary). If you need to loosen mucus, the best way to do it probably is to drink more fluids.

What about something to stop the cough? Most suppressants contain codeine or one of its derivatives, and they do stop a dry, irritating cough. The downside is their side effects, such as constipation and drowsiness. If your cough is loose, it's not a good idea to suppress it, because the cough is nature's way of getting rid of the phlegm.

THE BOTTOM LINE

There is some disagreement about these recommendations. Expectorants probably don't do much good, although everyone agrees that they can do no harm. As for suppressants, I think that if a dry, hacking cough is interfering with your sleep, you should take cough syrup. However, if the cough is already loose, a suppressant will prevent you from getting rid of mucus in your respiratory tract. First try the other time-honored alternatives, such as hot beverages and chicken soup, and keep the cough syrup handy just in case. If you weaken and do take a couple of teaspoons, don't worry about it. Just make sure you have a laxative handy and be prepared for a little drowsiness. ▪

COLON CANCER

Fiber *Does* Protect Against Colon Cancer

ABOUT 30 YEARS AGO, a British doctor named Denis Burkitt, working in Africa, made three interesting observations about the poor people living there: (a) they produced more feces than those in developed countries, (b) they ate much more fiber, and (c) they had a much lower incidence of colon cancer. He put these facts together and came up with the hypothesis that fiber in the diet protects against constipation and cancer of the bowel. The mechanism he suggested to explain fiber's beneficial effect was that it dilutes and absorbs cancer-causing agents and adds bulk to the stool, so these carcinogens are excreted more quickly. According to another theory, fiber decreases the quantity of bile acids excreted by the liver into the bowel thus reducing the irritation to its walls. Whichever reason you believe, you end up with fewer instances of bowel cancer.

For more than a quarter century, this relationship between fiber and bowel cancer remained dogma in this country. Breakfast food makers had a bonanza with it because grain (along with fruits and vegetables) is a major source of dietary fiber. Then in 1999, findings in the ongoing Nurses Study at Harvard, the source of many important epidemiological observations, apparently debunked the fiber-cancer link. Follow-up of more than 88,000 women over a 16-year period revealed that the incidence of colon cancer was not affected by the amount of fiber consumed. The following year, two other studies conducted over a 4-year period also failed to demonstrate any correlation between cancer and diets or supplements high in fiber. The theory linking the two has remained in limbo—until now.

■ HERE'S WHAT'S NEW

According to two major new studies published in *The Lancet* medical journal, one done in the United States and the other in Europe, the amount of fiber you consume makes a *big* difference in your vulnerability to colon tumors. The average daily fiber consumption in this country is about 16 grams a day; in Europe it's about 22 grams a day. (To give you some idea of what this means in practical terms, one slice of whole wheat bread contains 2 grams, a banana has 3 grams, an apple or a cup of brown rice contain 3.5 grams, a half cup of a fiber-rich cereal may have as much as 10 grams.)

The European research involved more than 500,000 people in 10 countries, and dwarfed all earlier studies. In the United States, the impact of fiber was evaluated among 3,600 men and women who'd previously had colon polyps (which often are precursors of cancer) and compared their outcome with that of about 34,000 healthy individuals. In both studies, the more fiber consumed, the lower the incidence of bowel cancer. In the American study, those who ate the most fiber (36 grams a day) had a 27 percent lower incidence of colon cancer than those who ate the least (12 grams a day). The European researchers obtained similar results. The subjects who ate 35 grams of fiber a day had a 40 percent lower rate of bowel cancer than those who consumed only 15 grams a day.

■ THE BOTTOM LINE

Any way you look at it, there is no downside to eating lots of fiber. It helps control weight; it makes for softer, more comfortable stools; and most important, it reduces the risk of colon cancer. Seems like a no-brainer to me. So, do yourself a favor, and enjoy a cup of a high-fiber grain cereal in the morning. Just be sure that if you decide to add more fiber to your diet, you do it gradually and drink a lot of water as well.

Don't Blush, Look Before You Flush!

COLON CANCER is a major killer, but it can be cured if detected early enough. Everyone should have a routine colonoscopy starting at age 50. If nothing is found, the test is usually repeated in 10 years; however, if polyps are detected in your initial colonoscopy or you have a strong family history of this malignancy, the test is done more frequently. Keep in mind that between tests it's important to report to your doctor any new abdominal signs or symptoms, changes in bowel habits, or the appearance of blood in your stool. Blood in the stool is not always easy to see, so ask for a fecal occult blood test, a little card on which you place a specimen to be analyzed for blood.

It's also wise to look at your own stool after every bowel movement. That's what the British medical establishment wants everyone to do, and to encourage people to do so, they've come up with the phrase, "Don't Blush, Look Before You Flush."

■ HERE'S WHAT'S NEW

British gastroenterologists have pointed out a surprising problem with this advice—the use of toilet disinfectants, most of which are bright blue. These solutions make it more difficult to tell if there's blood in the stool. So they have embarked on a campaign in the

United Kingdom to discourage manufacturers from coloring their toilet disinfectants. We should, too.

■ THE BOTTOM LINE

I suggest you stop using colored toilet disinfectants. Instead, look carefully at the stool and the color of the water in the toilet bowl to detect the presence of blood. It can save your life.

Prevent Colon Cancer from Recurring—
Or Even Happening

SUPPOSE YOU'RE A CANCER SURVIVOR, one of the lucky ones. Your colon (or colorectal) cancer was discovered in time and removed. But you aren't free and clear because you know you're more likely to develop cancer again than someone who's never had the problem. This is true especially if you developed the cancer before you turned 60 or you also have chronic inflammatory bowel disease. So your doctor has advised you to have another colonoscopy in a year, looking not only for a recurrence of the cancer itself, but for the presence of new polyps that sometimes become malignant later on. You were told also to look carefully at every stool you produce for evidence of blood.

There's lots more you can do to reduce the risk of another colorectal cancer. For starters, eat less red meat and have at least five to seven servings a day of fruits and vegetables, as well as other foods from plant sources (beans, grain products, and pasta). Exercise regularly, too, and don't just watch your weight, do something about it if you're overweight. You may think that smoking is bad for only the lungs. The fact is smokers are 30 percent to 40 percent more likely to die of colon cancer than nonsmokers. Finally, because booze is a risk factor of bowel cancer, limit your intake to one or two drinks per day.

You were lucky the first time around. Don't tempt fate now by failing to heed this advice—as well as what follows.

■ HERE'S WHAT'S NEW

Researchers at the University of North Carolina in Chapel Hill studied 635 subjects with a history of colorectal cancer. They found that those who took an adult dose of aspirin (325 milligrams) every day had a 35 percent lower risk of developing colon polyps than subjects who were given a placebo. That's important because although only 5 to 10 percent of colon polyps become cancerous in individuals with no previous history, that risk is greatly increased if you've previously had a malignancy of the colon. Other studies have shown that nonsteroidal anti-inflammatories (NSAIDs) also reduce the risk of colon cancer, presumably because of the same anti-inflammatory effect as aspirin.

And, there's even more you can do if you have a history of colon cancer. If, for any reason, you can't take aspirin (either because you're allergic to it or it makes you bleed from the stomach), ask your doctor about calcium supplements. They, too, can prevent polyp formation. Even if you have no problem with aspirin, take the calcium anyway. You might as well protect your bones along with your bowel!

Here's even more good news! This time it's tea, one of the most widely consumed and inexpensive beverages in the world. Studies funded by the National Cancer Institute have determined that drinking three cups of green or white tea every day can prevent certain colon cancers (black tea does not appear to be as protective). Researchers believe that the beneficial action of these types of tea stems from the polyphenols they contain. Tea is especially effective when combined with an anti-inflammatory drug.

■ THE BOTTOM LINE

Fortunately, there is a great deal you can do to prevent recurrence of colon cancer, and even its first appearance. Lifestyle and diet are important. Adding aspirin or one of the NSAIDs like Advil (ibuprofen) is important, as are calcium and the daily consumption of green or white tea.

However, none of these steps is a substitute for regular screening—this includes annual screening of stool specimens for traces of blood not visible to the human eye. You should have a colonoscopy every year if you've already had a colon cancer.

For someone without a previous history of colon polyps or cancer, I recommend a colonoscopy at age 50 with follow-ups at appropriate intervals based on what was found and details of your family history. Routinely, your doctor should request a flexible sigmoidoscopy (a procedure that examines part of the colon) every 5 years and a colonoscopy (that looks at the entire colon) every 10 years.

WHAT THE DOCTOR ORDERED?

BETA-CAROTENE: GOOD AND BAD

■ Everyone knows that fruits and vegetable are good for the heart and that they also reduce the risk of cancer. Carotenes are considered to be prime among the many ingredients that afford these health benefits. There are several different kinds of carotenes, the best known of which is beta-carotene. It is extracted from fruits and vegetables and put into capsules either alone or combined with other vitamins. Presumably, the logic for doing so is that if fruits and vegetables are good for you, then high doses of one of their main ingredients should be, too.

This assumption led to a famous study in Finland in the 1990s. Its purpose was to see whether taking beta-carotene would reduce the incidence of lung cancer in heavy cigarette smokers.

The research project looked at 29,000 male subjects who were randomly assigned to one of four regimens: 1) beta-carotene alone, 2) beta-carotene and vitamin E, 3) vitamin E alone, or 4) a placebo. Neither the researchers nor the participants in the study knew who was getting what. After 8 years, researchers evaluated the findings. Guess what? Those subjects who received the beta-carotene had an 18 percent *higher* incidence of lung cancer and an 8 percent higher death rate from all causes than the "unlucky" controls who did not.

That destroyed the myth of beta-carotene, at least in my mind, although it continued to be advertised as a health panacea and sold in health food stores everywhere.

HERE'S WHAT'S NEW

A 2003 study at the Dartmouth Medical School looked once more at the impact of beta-carotene on cancer. The new target was colon polyps (which sometimes lead to colorectal cancer). As was the case with lung cancer, the researchers found that participants who received the usual daily 25-milligram dose of beta-carotene *and who smoked cigarettes or had more than one alcoholic drink a day or both* were at *twice* the risk of developing recurrent adenomas (polyps) when compared with the controls.

But here's the big news. The beta-carotene actually *reduced* the risk of these polyps by 44 percent in *nonsmokers and nondrinkers*. There appears to be something in tobacco and alcohol that interacts unfavorably with beta-carotene.

THE BOTTOM LINE

Fruits and vegetables are good for you. All their ingredients *working together* guard your health against various diseases. However, the effect of any single component is unpredictable. Beta-carotene is a case in point. It seems from at least two studies that when this supplement is given to drinkers or smokers, it *increases* the risk of certain cancers; however it appears to protect against colon polyps in people who neither drink nor smoke.

So here's my advice. Eat all the whole fruits and vegetables you can—at least 6 to 8 servings a day. If you can't manage that, take a daily 25-milligram dose of beta-carotene, but only *if you neither drink nor smoke*. (Avoid it if you're a smoker or drinker, even a social one.) Also, remember that beta-carotene is present in many multivitamins, so look at the label on the one you're taking. ▪

DEEP VEIN THROMBOSIS

Take Blood Thinners for How Long?

EACH YEAR, an estimated two million Americans develop deep vein thrombosis (DVT), in which one or more blood clots form in the veins deep inside the leg. Signs and symptoms of DVT include pain and swelling of the leg, distention of the superficial veins just under the skin, as well as reddish blue discoloration and increased warmth of the skin.

Anyone older than age 60 is especially vulnerable to DVT (but it can occur at any age), and the risk increases as you get older. However, the greatest danger is for anyone who has been confined to bed for 3 or more days for any reason—chronic illness, an injury, or surgery; women who take the estrogen-containing birth control pill and also smoke; and anyone with heart or lung failure or a genetic predisposition to clotting.

Other risk factors include obesity, varicose veins, history of a previous clot, certain congenital heart defects, and hormone replacement therapy in postmenopausal women. DVT also has been referred to as the "economy class syndrome" because it commonly occurs after a person has sat for hours on a plane in a small seat with little legroom.

The list of risks is long, but if any of the above situations applies to you, suspect DVT if you develop unexplained pain or tenderness in your legs.

DVT is a serious illness on two counts. If the clots are large enough, they can obstruct the veins so that blood backs up and causes the legs to swell. More important, the clots themselves can break up and their fragments can travel along the body's network of veins, ending up in the lungs and blocking one more pulmonary arteries. This complication, called pulmonary embolism, is a major cause of death in the United States where it is responsible for an estimated 60,000 deaths every year.

These deaths are preventable if the DVT is properly diagnosed and treated immediately. Unfortunately, the classic symptoms often go unrecognized, undetected, and not reported to the doctor.

So always think of a pulmonary embolism, especially if you have been diagnosed with DVT and you experience any of the following signs or symptoms: chest pain that is worse when you take a deep breath, the onset of cough without any cold or flu symptoms, or the presence of blood in the sputum. These signs and symptoms should raise the red flag of a pulmonary embolus not only if you have obvious DVT but also if you've recently been on a long trip, had surgery, or been confined to bed for 3 days or more.

DVT, with or without a pulmonary embolus, should be treated by "thinning" the blood with anticoagulants as soon as the diagnosis is made. Two drugs usually are started simultaneously: heparin and Coumadin (warfarin). Heparin acts immediately, is given by injection under the skin or into a vein, and usually needs to be continued for 5 to 7 days. Warfarin is administered orally, acts in a different way, and takes a few days to reach effective levels in the blood. After it does so, the heparin is stopped and the warfarin is continued alone.

For years, doctors have debated how long to continue warfarin therapy in patients with DVT, pulmonary embolus, or both. Staying on this medication indefinitely requires checking your blood every few weeks to see that the "thinning" level is optimal, or as Goldilocks would have put it, "Neither too thick nor too thin, but just right." However, a greater drawback of long-term anticoagulant use is the danger of internal bleeding. Such bleeding can occur spontaneously or after an injury. The hazard is especially great in older people who are prone to falling, making them vulnerable to brain hemorrhage. Also, one has to be careful about taking warfarin along with other drugs, such as aspirin, any of the NSAIDs, and even such widely used herbs as garlic and gingko. These combinations can increase the risk of bleeding.

■ HERE'S WHAT'S NEW

The question of how long to continue anticoagulation was addressed in an important study involving hundreds of patients with DVT. Here are its important conclusions and recommendations.

If you've had DVT with or without a pulmonary embolus, you should be treated with heparin and warfarin together immediately. The heparin should be continued for 5 to 7 days and the warfarin for anywhere between 6 and 12 months. If whatever caused the DVT is no longer active and you're no longer at risk for it acting up, you may then stop the warfarin as far as this particular episode of DVT is concerned. However, there is a 5 to 10 percent risk of another clot forming during the next 12 months. So try not expose yourself during that interval to any of the risk factors for DVT.

Beyond the first year after discontinuing the anticoagulants, the risk of clots recurring drops to only 1 to 2 percent per year. No matter how long you continue the warfarin after your DVT—5 years, 10 years, or even longer—once you stop it, you will still have this "catch-up" risk of 5 to 10 percent for 1 year. That's presumably because of the body's reaction to going off warfarin—a kind of rebound phenomenon.

Some people (and their doctors) will decide not to take the risk and will opt to continue to take the anticoagulant indefinitely. As long as you do so, you'll be protected against DVT and embolism. The downside of staying on the warfarin is the risk of bleeding and the fact that you have the same 5 to 10 percent chance for DVT whenever you stop the therapy. Strange, but true!

■ THE BOTTOM LINE

Treating DVT with anticoagulants immediately after it's diagnosed can prevent the potentially lethal complication of a blood clot to the lung. After the original risk factors that cause the DVT are no longer present, this therapy is usually discontinued at some point. There's a 5 to 10 percent chance of another DVT occurring during the following 12 months. After that, the risk drops to between 1 and 2 percent. If you have a chronic disorder, such as heart failure or serious lung disease, it makes sense to continue long-term warfarin therapy (just as you would for an artificial heart valve or chronic atrial fibrillation). Otherwise you may want to take your chances and discontinue the warfarin after 1 year.

DEPRESSION

Prozac for Kids?

OVERALL, 6 percent of children and teenagers in the United States take medication for depression, attention-deficit hyperactivity disorder, and other behavioral and emotional problems. Many of the drugs, especially the antidepressants, are the same as those given to adults, but have not been approved by the FDA for children. The best known of these is Prozac (fluoxetine).

■ HERE'S WHAT'S NEW

After reviewing all available data, the FDA now believes that there is enough evidence of Prozac's effectiveness to warrant its approval for treating depression in children older than age 7. However, parents of these children should know that Prozac can have such adverse effects as nausea, fatigue, dizziness, difficulty concentrating, and nervousness. And they should bear in mind an additional adverse effect unique to kids and teenagers: They may grow more slowly and gain less weight. Researchers are trying to determine whether these children eventually catch up.

What's true for Prozac doesn't necessarily apply to other drugs classified as selective serotonin reuptake inhibitors (SSRIs). For example, the FDA has ruled that Paxil (paroxetine) should not be taken by anyone younger than age 18 because it is associated with a possible increased risk of suicidal impulses.

■ THE BOTTOM LINE

Depressed children and teenagers may be treated with Prozac if their doctors believe the symptoms are serious enough to justify it. Such therapy is safe, according to the FDA. But if your child is taking Prozac, make sure a pediatrician closely monitors his or her weight and growth.

WHAT THE DOCTOR ORDERED?

ANTIDEPRESSANTS—ANOTHER CAUSE OF UPPER GASTROINTESTINAL BLEEDING ■ As we get older, blood vessels in the stomach and, to a lesser extent, the small intestine, become more vulnerable to irritation and bleeding. That's why older people who regularly take aspirin and/or a nonsteroidal anti-inflammatory drug (NSAID), such as Motrin (ibuprofen) or Aleve (naproxen), have a higher incidence of these complications.

HERE'S WHAT'S NEW

Researchers in Denmark have found that the selective serotonin reuptake inhibitors (SSRIs), the newest antidepressants, are associated with a significantly increased risk of gastrointestinal bleeding. These drugs, the best known of which are Prozac (fluoxetine) and Paxil (paroxetine) but there are many others, are widely used throughout the world. A study of 26,000 patients taking SSRIs concluded that these drugs caused more stomach bleeding when taken alone and were especially risky when combined with either aspirin (5.2 times the incidence of bleeding) or an NSAID (12.2 times the risk). The researchers believe that some interaction between the antidepressant and the blood platelets accounts for this adverse effect.

THE BOTTOM LINE

If you're taking an SSRI, watch for evidence of bleeding from your intestinal tract—especially if you're older and also taking aspirin or an NSAID. Look for black stools, which indicate the presence of blood, and have them routinely checked by your doctor. (Note that iron supplements also can make stools black.) Report any stomach pain to your doctor; there are other categories of antidepressants that can be prescribed. ▪

Are Antidepressants Safe during Pregnancy and Breastfeeding?

AS MANY AS 15 PERCENT of women of childbearing age are chronically depressed. Some even become suicidal. When such depression leads to alcohol or drugs, it can have especially serious long-term consequences for a woman and her baby during pregnancy or breastfeeding.

Normal brain function depends on an adequate supply of certain chemical "messengers," such as serotonin and norepinephrine, which transmit signals from one part of the brain to another. People with major depression have lower levels of these substances. The newest antidepressants, called selective serotonin reuptake inhibitors (SSRIs) have dramatically improved the mood and quality of life for thousands of depression sufferers by raising serotonin levels in the brain.

Will pregnant women and nursing mothers who need these drugs harm their children by taking them?

■ HERE'S WHAT'S NEW

Even though these drugs can be passed to the fetus via the bloodstream, research indicates that the newer SSRIs such as Prozac (fluoxetine), Paxil (paroxetine), Zoloft (sertraline), Celexa (citalopram), and Effexor (venlafaxine), do not increase fetal risk of major birth defects or death. However, to avoid withdrawal symptoms in newborns, some doctors recommend that these medications be tapered or discontinued 10 to 14 days before the patient's due date.

Doctors at the University of Bergen in Norway analyzed breast milk from 23 women who were taking an SSRI for depression while breastfeeding their babies. Blood samples from the mothers and children revealed that the drug was not present in breast milk or the babies' blood in appreciable amounts. The researchers conclude that these antidepressants are safe to take while nursing. In fact, they are especially useful in treating postpartum depression.

■ THE BOTTOM LINE

If you're seriously depressed while pregnant or breastfeeding, you may benefit from taking an SSRI at the lowest effective dose. But as with any medication, it's important for your doctor to monitor its use. You should also receive appropriate counseling and emotional support. Although some SSRIs, such as Prozac, may result in higher blood levels in the nursing infants than others (Paxil and Zoloft have the lowest concentrations in breast milk), none are high enough to harm the child.

DIABETES

You *Can* Prevent Diabetes

MONUMENTAL PROGRESS IS BEING MADE in virtually every field of medicine. Vaccines, diagnostic equipment, surgical techniques, heart disease and cancer treatments . . . you name it, scientists are hard at work making it better. Advances in diabetes—ways to prevent it and better, easier ways to treat it—are also at the forefront of research.

Let's review the basics of this disease. There are two kinds of diabetes. As far as we know, they have totally different causes. Type 1 affects youngsters and is caused by the destruction of the cells in the pancreas that make insulin, a hormone that regulates glucose levels in the blood. The body's own immune system is responsible for this destruction, mistaking these cells for "enemy invaders." Type 1 diabetes falls into the autoimmune category of diseases. Up to now, such diseases have not been preventable. However, new research described in this chapter may change all that.

Type 2 (or adult-onset) diabetes accounts for 90 percent of cases.

People with type 2 diabetes are able to make insulin, but the cells don't allow the hormone to enter them and burn the glucose.

The end result in both types of diabetes is elevated blood glucose levels with all its consequences, the most important of which are generalized disease of blood vessels, as well as neurologic abnormalities.

Type 2 diabetes can be prevented through weight loss, diet, and exercise. Diet is especially important and should include whole grains (as opposed to refined grains such as those in white bread). Whole grains increase the efficiency of insulin so that less is required to process glucose.

■ HERE'S WHAT'S NEW

Scientists have discovered an antibody that can stop the abnormal autoimmune response in type 1 diabetes from destroying the insulin-producing cells. This research is still in its early stages.

Researchers also are looking into another theory that type 1 diabetes is caused by an abnormal response of the body to some viral infection during childhood. If this is true, it may be possible to develop a vaccine that could prevent both the infection and the diabetes.

With regard to staving off type 2 diabetes, two drugs have been found useful. Glucophage (metformin), a prescription drug that limits the amount of glucose made by the liver, can help prevent diabetes in people who are obese, who have borderline blood glucose levels, and who have a family history of diabetes. However, it is not as effective as weight loss, diet, and exercise.

Xenical (orlistat) is another drug useful in preventing type 2 diabetes in those especially vulnerable to the disease. It works by binding with the fat you've eaten after it reaches the stomach. As a result, this fat is not absorbed and passes out of the body in the stool along with the orlistat. Recent studies have shown that orlistat may play an important role in preventing heart disease, especially in diabetics, by reducing cholesterol levels and body weight.

■ THE BOTTOM LINE

If you're overweight and worried about developing diabetes because of a bad family history, or if you have a borderline blood glucose level, you can reduce your risk by getting lots of exercise, losing weight, and adding whole grains and nuts to your diet. Also, ask your doctor about taking metformin and orlistat, both of which also may prevent the onset of this disease. If you decide to use orlistat, also be sure to take vitamins A, D, E, and K because these fat-soluble vitamins are excreted along with the dietary fat bound by orlistat.

A New Diabetes Home Test

THE SINGLE MOST IMPORTANT THING people with diabetes can do to reduce the complications of their disease is to keep their blood glucose levels as close to normal as possible. The easiest way to do so is to monitor blood sugar frequently using the fingerstick method. However, those results only tell you what's happening at that particular moment. Normal blood glucose at 2 P.M. does not necessarily indicate that it will remain normal the rest of the day—let alone the week.

To help patients control their blood glucose levels more efficiently over the long-term, doctors use another blood test that measures glycolated hemoglobin (also referred to as hemoglobin A1c) about every 6 weeks. It reflects the average blood glucose level during the previous 6 to 12 weeks. Diabetics treated with insulin should have this test at least four times a year and more frequently if their blood glucose level is difficult to control. Until now the glycolated hemoglobin test could only be done in the doctor's office.

■ HERE'S WHAT'S NEW

The FDA has approved Metrika A1c, the first over-the-counter test you can use to measure glycolated hemoglobin levels at home. It gives you results immediately.

■ THE BOTTOM LINE

I suggest that all diabetics take advantage of this test. Medicare will pay for it as it does for most other routine diabetic supplies. Continue to use the fingerstick method to check your blood glucose level during the day, but test your hemoglobin A1c every 6 weeks for a better idea of how you're managing your diabetes over the long-term.

No More Pins and Needles?

REGULAR MONITORING of the blood glucose level is the best way to keep diabetes under control and the ravages of the disease at bay. This means frequent finger pricking to obtain a drop of blood for analysis. Most diabetics become resigned to it yet long for some device to do it noninvasively. Doctors also have been looking for alternatives to injectable insulin.

■ HERE'S WHAT'S NEW

The G2 Biographer from GlucoWatch can determine blood glucose levels noninvasively. Worn on the wrist, the device emits a low-level electric current that pulls glucose through the skin. It measures your glucose level over 13 hours, and sends an alarm if the reading is abnormal. The G2 can determine trends in your blood glucose to alert you to an impending significant drop. You can then adjust your insulin dosage and diet accordingly. Doing it at bedtime is especially useful for predicting if your blood glucose level may drop while you're asleep.

This device is not a substitute for the conventional skin prick that tells you your blood glucose level at a particular point in time. The G2 Biographer is meant to augment, rather than replace, conventional testing. (There's an equally interesting device already on the market in Europe that measures the blood glucose level using infrared rays directed at the skin. It is not yet available here.)

Considerable progress also has been made with regard to alternatives to injected insulin, for example:

Insulin pills. Several pills and capsules now being tested can deliver insulin into the bloodstream within 20 minutes. The most recent experiments indicate that these preparations lower blood glucose levels in patients with type 2 diabetes as effectively as injected insulin. Although they are not yet on the market, you can look forward to their availability in the near future.

Insulin spray. The insulin is delivered via inhalers similar to those used by asthmatics. The dose is absorbed by mucous membranes in the cheeks, tongue, and throat. The spray has been shown to work, and I also predict its early approval.

Insulin patch. An electronic adhesive patch is first applied to the skin, where it painlessly vaporizes the cells on the surface, creating microscopic pores. Then a small insulin-coated patch is placed on the area, and the insulin is steadily absorbed through the openings for 12 hours. This is also an exciting prospect.

■ THE BOTTOM LINE

You can now buy a "watch" to wear on your wrist that can give you a good idea of how well your insulin dosage is correcting your blood glucose level. It is not as useful for assessing your glucose level here and now, for which purpose you still need to prick your finger. You can look forward to taking your insulin by the oral, inhaled, or topical insulin delivery instead of by injection before too long.

A Fishy Solution

DIABETES LEADS to several life-threatening vascular complications—heart disease and stroke among them. Diabetics, regardless of whether they require insulin, must control their glucose levels and the other risk factors for vascular disease, such as high blood

pressure, obesity, high cholesterol levels, physical inactivity, and tobacco use.

■ HERE'S WHAT'S NEW

Researchers from the Harvard School of Public Health and other
Boston institutions studied more than 5,000 women with type 2
(adult-onset) diabetes enrolled in the famous Nurses Health Study.
Their purpose was to determine the impact of consuming the omega-
3 fatty acids present in cold-water, oily fish on the complications of
coronary heart disease and sudden death among diabetics. No subject
evaluated had either heart disease or cancer at the onset of the study.
During the next 16 years, those diabetic women who ate this type of
fish more than five times a week enjoyed a 64 percent reduction in
heart attacks and overall mortality. Eating fish only one to three times
a month led to a 30 percent lower risk of heart disease and death from
any cause. Eating it once a week resulted in a 40 percent reduction.

■ THE BOTTOM LINE

Besides controlling all other risk factors for vascular disease, every
diabetic should make a point of eating fish whenever possible—at
least once a week, and ideally, five or more times a week. Fish rich in
the omega-3 fatty acids include mackerel, sardines, tuna, and salmon.
(Pregnant women should not eat mackerel, tuna, tilefish, swordfish,
and shark because of their high mercury content—although canned
fish is safe.)

You can also buy omega-3 fatty acids in capsule form. Omega
Brite, Solgar, and TwinLabs are reliable brands.

The Promise of a Better Quality of Life

A DIABETIC'S LIFE is much better these days than it used to be.
Home monitors for testing blood glucose levels have resulted in

fewer attacks of low or high blood glucose levels, both of which once frequently caused coma. Years ago, when I worked as a resident in the emergency department, such cases were common. Oral medications as well as new forms of insulin have made blood glucose control smoother, allowing for fewer peaks and valleys. But most important are the new discoveries on the horizon that promise to further reduce the complications of this disease and possibly even cure it.

■ HERE'S WHAT'S NEW

Perhaps the most exciting news on the diabetes front is the result of work pioneered in Canada, where researchers in 1999 harvested insulin-producing pancreatic islet cells from fresh cadavers and transplanted them into patients with type 1 diabetes. The cells were injected into the blood and traveled to the liver, where they continued to make insulin.

Initial results of the treatment were extremely promising. All of the first seven patients treated were able to discontinue insulin injections or pumps and enjoy normal blood glucose levels.

Currently, researchers are continuing to evaluate 36 more patients who were treated with these islet cell injections. Results to date have varied depending on where the procedures were done. For example, 90 percent of patients treated in Canada by the original researchers, as well as in a couple of American centers, no longer require insulin injections. However, in other locales, the success rate is only 3 out of 13. Hopefully, as doctors gain experience with this technique, the results will be more uniformly successful.

Although this concept is exciting and promising, it is not without inherent problems. Harvesting insulin-producing cells from a cadaver pancreas is difficult and time-consuming. These islet cells comprise only 3 to 4 percent of the million cells in each pancreas. They must be carefully "teased" from each fresh organ in a procedure that takes about 6 hours, and two organs usually are required to generate enough cells for one patient. Furthermore, after the cells are transferred, the recipient must take several anti-rejection drugs indefinitely, and these can have some adverse effects.

In other news about breakthrough treatment for diabetes, scientists at the Centre for Regenerative Medicine at the University of Bath in the United Kingdom have developed a genetic-engineering process to transform human liver cells so that they can make insulin. They are now looking to see whether these new cells can respond to fluctuating glucose levels in the blood. In the human body, when the blood glucose level is normal, the cells that make insulin reduce its production. When the blood glucose level rises, more insulin is made. The question is whether these genetically engineered insulin-producing liver cells can respond in this way. This entire project is early in its development, but it gives you some idea of the ingenious thoughts that occur to dedicated researchers.

There also may be a future in diabetes for stem-cell transplantation, transforming immature cells into insulin-producing tissues. This is probably the hottest area of research today for virtually every disease. Primitive cells that have not yet assumed an identity, derived either from embryos or normal bone marrow, are being introduced into damaged tissue in the hope they will grow to become—and ultimately replace—the cells that have been destroyed. To date, such stem cells have been injected into hearts whose muscle has been destroyed by heart attack as well as into brains that have been damaged by stroke or affected by diseases such as Parkinson's. There is already considerable evidence that these stem cells assume the identity of whatever tissue has been destroyed and needs to be replaced. Cells that make insulin will no doubt also be targeted.

■ THE BOTTOM LINE

If you have type 1 diabetes and your disease is difficult to control and has begun to damage other organs such as the kidney or the eyes, it's worth looking into islet cell transfer. The results have been encouraging, and it's only a matter of time until researchers refine the technique.

Although genetic engineering and stem-cell transplantation are still further away, they look promising. The importance of my message to you is that this research is taking place and that a cure is indeed on the horizon.

WHAT THE DOCTOR ORDERED?

MULTIVITAMINS FOR DIABETICS WITH COLDS ■ Multivitamins are the epitome of the "quick fix" for which Americans are always looking. What harm, patients ask me, is there in popping one or two multivitamins every morning with breakfast? They aren't really drugs, are they? Multivitamins seduce so many of us mainly because they contain all the good things in the healthy foods that many of us never get around to eating—such as fruits and vegetables. As a result, at least 40 percent of Americans (who can afford them) take multivitamins.

Do multivitamins really do any good, or is it just wishful thinking? Several studies have attempted to answer that question. Unfortunately, the results are inconclusive because the goals of the studies are never quite clear. What do you look for when trying to decide whether a multivitamin is doing you any good? How you feel? That's pretty vague—vulnerable to many variables. And who can wait a lifetime to see whether the vitamins help people to live longer or better? So the studies' "end points"—that is, the things researchers measure to decide whether a given therapy is having an effect—are difficult to establish as far as multivitamin use is concerned.

Personally, I believe multivitamins are good (and actually necessary) for growing children, anyone who goes through life in and out of various crash diets, the elderly who live alone and whose nutrition may be compromised, and people who have documented nutritional deficiencies, such as those in developing countries.

HERE'S WHAT'S NEW

Doctors at the Carolinas Medical Center in Charlotte, North Carolina, undertook a research project that had a specific, well-defined goal: to determine whether an over-the-counter multivitamin had any effect on the immune systems (and therefore the resistance) of people with adult-onset, type 2 diabetes who were at least 45 years old. Such patients are generally more susceptible to viral and bacterial infections. Would the supplement protect them?

The answer in this small study was a resounding yes! The researchers found that only 17 percent of the diabetics who took a multivitamin developed a cold or other infection, while 93 percent of those receiving a placebo got sick. In a control group of subjects who were not diabetic, the supplement had no effect. In other words, it protected only the diabetics.

Why the difference in the responses of the diabetics versus the control group? One possible explanation is that the elevated blood glucose level in diabetics interferes with the action of infection-fighting white blood cells, preventing them from killing bacteria and viruses as effectively. Another theory is that because diabetics urinate more frequently and copiously (in order for the body to eliminate excess glucose), they may excrete too much of certain substances that are thought to strengthen the immune system, including zinc and selenium. (People with diabetes have never been shown to be deficient in these chemicals.) The study findings are interesting regardless of how they're explained.

THE BOTTOM LINE

This small study will surely be repeated. In the meantime, if you have type 2 diabetes, there's no harm in taking a multivitamin once or twice a day. In fact, why not do so even if you have type 1 diabetes? Just make sure that the preparation contains some selenium and zinc, because they seem to be the major players. ▪

ECZEMA

Mom Could Have Prevented You
from Getting It

ECZEMA, OR ATOPIC DERMATITIS, is a chronic skin condition that affects about 10 percent of infants and children and 3 percent of adults in this country. You're more likely to have it if a close relative does too or suffers from hay fever, food allergies, or asthma. However, 20 percent of eczema patients have no such family history.

Teenagers and adults with eczema usually have dry, itchy skin, with reddish brown or gray, scaly, and thickened patches that appear mostly on the hands and feet and are easily irritated. In infants, the rash usually starts out on the face and scalp and is apt to ooze and crust. Once the baby begins crawling, exposed areas (such as the knees, elbows, ankles, wrists, and hands) also become affected.

Eczema generally improves by age 25, but it persists throughout life in 50 percent of cases. Itching is the most troublesome and common complaint with eczema in all age groups. (Incidentally, if you have a history of this kind of condition, you shouldn't have a smallpox vaccination—see page 236.)

Treatment of eczema basically involves the use of topical medications—cortisone creams, ointments, lotions, and sometimes tars. Oral antihistamines can alleviate the itch. Antibiotics may be necessary if the skin is infected. Dermatologists sometimes recommend treatment with ultraviolet light if the condition is severe. (Avoid oral steroids unless absolutely necessary. Their long-term use can result in a host of complications ranging from impaired immune response to gastric bleeding and osteoporosis.)

A new class of medications called immunomodulators represents a major breakthrough in therapy for severe atopic dermatitis. These drugs, usually taken orally by transplant patients to help prevent organ rejection, can also clear up severe eczema when applied topically for long periods of time. The flagship drug in this category is Prograf (tacrolimus).

Patients with atopic dermatitis must learn how to take care of their skin. Food allergies play a role in up to 30 percent of cases, so avoid foods that you know make it worse. Some substances in the environment—soaps, detergents, perfumes, cosmetics, even smoke—can aggravate the rash either through physical or respiratory contact. Neither skin testing nor allergy "shots" are usually of much help, so don't waste your time and money on them unless your dermatologist specifically recommends them.

▪ HERE'S WHAT'S NEW

As noted on page 24, kids raised in a compulsively clean environment are more likely to develop asthma and other allergic conditions, at least during infancy. It seems that getting rid of every vestige of dust, mites, and other allergenic substances in the home doesn't give the body's immune system a chance (or a reason) to tool up. Unprovoked, our defenses slumber, then when attacked by the real thing, all hell breaks loose in the form of allergic reactions of one kind or another.

Acting on the assumption that, like asthma and other allergic responses, eczema may also result from decreased bacterial exposure early in life, researchers decided to give pregnant women a harmless infection that would activate their immune system and protect the fetus from atopic dermatitis. They used a "probiotic" (the opposite of an "antibiotic") called lactobacillus. Doctors prescribe this innocuous organism for patients on long-term antibiotic therapy that kills good bacteria along with the harmful ones. This leaves the field wide open for invasion by yeast and other organisms. Lactobacillus (present in some foods and many supplements) introduces into the environment harmless bacteria that reduce the growth of yeast and other organisms.

This study confirmed the findings from an earlier one, showing that children born to mothers who were given lactobacillus just before delivery were 40 percent less likely to develop atopic dermatitis. This protection lasted at least until the child was 4 years old. (Note, however, that this beneficial effect protected the child only against atopic dermatitis, not asthma or other allergies.)

■ THE BOTTOM LINE

Atopic dermatitis is a lousy skin condition to have. The only good thing about it is the excuse it provides for you not getting the optional smallpox vaccine. Although there are many ways to treat this disorder, you're better off preventing it. If you're pregnant—and especially if you have a family history of allergy or atopic dermatitis—why not eat some yogurt (containing lactobacillus) or get your lactobacillus some other way (such as a tablet) a few days before your delivery date? Studies suggest that this may reduce the risk of atopic dermatitis. Try it. You may like it.

EYE PROBLEMS

Keep Your Eyes on Fish

THE EYES ARE VULNERABLE to several unpleasant changes as we grow older. Among the most common are cataracts (easily removed by surgery), macular degeneration (commonly resulting in blindness because treatment is not very successful), and dry eyes (uncomfortable, but manageable).

Macular degeneration is the leading cause of significant permanent vision loss in this country—and about two million people can't see well because of it. Nearly all are older than age 65, most have light-colored eyes, and Caucasians are especially vulnerable. The incidence is expected to triple by the year 2020, as the population ages. About 165,000 new cases develop every year, around 16,000 of which result in blindness.

The macula is a tiny area in the middle of the retina, situated in the back of the eye. When the cells in the macula degenerate, you have trouble seeing what is straight ahead of you and colors may appear dull. However, because the rest of the retina is not usually affected, you can still see out of the sides of the eyes, though not straight ahead. Now you know why some of your older friends always sit beside the TV and not in front of it.

Risk factors for macular degeneration are pollution, a high-fat diet sparse in fruits and vegetables, cigarette smoking, and a lifetime of excessive, unprotected exposure to bright sunlight. The most effective strategy for preventing macular degeneration is to limit your exposure to these risks. Some evidence does suggest that zinc supplements (80 milligrams a day) may also help prevent macular degeneration.

Dry eye syndrome affects over 10 million Americans. This disorder is usually caused by a decrease in the amount of oil in the tears that lubricate the eyes. As a result, the tears evaporate much more quickly and impair vision by leaving the cornea (the outermost layer of the eyes) abnormally dry and more easily scarred.

Dry eye syndrome is basically a complication of aging. As we grow older, our bodies produce less oil—60 percent less at age 65 than at age 18. This decrease is more pronounced in women, who tend to have drier skin than men. Besides age, other factors also contribute to dry eye syndrome. These include living in a hot, dry, windy climate or at high altitudes; being continuously exposed to air-conditioning or cigarette smoke; and working long hours on a computer. Contact lenses also may be responsible because they can absorb tears and cause proteins to form on the surface of the lens. Low thyroid function, vitamin A deficiency, Parkinson's disease, and certain medications can also cause dryness, as can low estrogen levels after menopause. The autoimmune disorder called Sjögren's syndrome is also characterized by dry eyes.

■ HERE'S WHAT'S NEW

Two interesting recent research findings may significantly reduce the incidence of macular degeneration and dry eyes. With regard to macular degeneration, researchers at the National Eye Institute analyzed dietary data from more than 4,500 men and women ages 60 to 80. Those who regularly ate fish more than twice a week were half as likely to develop macular degeneration as those who ate no fish at all. Consuming more than one portion of broiled or baked fish a week lowered the risk by one-third.

The researchers believe that a component of fish oil, the omega-3 fatty acid called docosahexanoic acid (DHA), builds up in the eye near the light-sensing nerve cells of the macula and may prevent their deterioration. Another report, this one from the Brigham and Women's Hospital in Boston, debunked a popularly held belief that beta-carotene supplements help prevent macular degeneration. More than 22,000 men followed for 12 years, half of whom were given such supplements, showed no reduction in the incidence of macular degeneration.

A diet rich in fish can also benefit dry eye syndrome. Harvard researchers analyzed data from more than 32,000 female health professionals in their Women's Health Study and found that those who consumed the most fish (and therefore the highest amount of omega-3 fatty acids) were least likely to have dry eye syndrome. This was especially true among those women who ate the most fatty fish. Two to four servings of tuna a week resulted in an 18 percent reduction in the incidence of dry eye syndrome than did a lesser amount. Five or six 4-ounce servings a week lowered the risk by 66 percent!

■ THE BOTTOM LINE

This book is replete with examples of the many ways fish is good for you. The omega-3 fatty acids fish contain lower blood pressure and cholesterol, and reduce the "clottability" of the blood. Add to all this the prevention of both a major cause of blindness in the United States as well as an unpleasant ocular condition, and you have a real winner. (Pregnant women should avoid mackerel, tuna, tilefish, swordfish, and shark because of their high mercury levels. Canned fish is safe.)

If you don't enjoy eating fish, you can buy omega-3 fatty acids in capsule form. But be sure to purchase a well-known brand, such as Omega Brite, Solgar, TwinLabs, and others. Unless properly made, the oil can become rancid.

Look for the Safest Glaucoma Treatment

GLAUCOMA IS A DISORDER of the eye in which the pressure of the fluid it contains is increased and eventually damages the ocular nerve. Glaucoma affects at least three million people in the United States—half of whom are unaware of it until their vision becomes impaired. The disorder is the second leading cause of blindness in this country, accounting for 12 percent of all cases.

Tissues surrounding the lens of a healthy eye continuously produce a clear liquid called aqueous humor that keep its interior moist. (This liquid has nothing to do with tears, which are made outside the eye with the purpose of preventing the outer surface from drying.) Aqueous humor flows in and out of the eye through the pupil, and is reabsorbed into the bloodstream through a meshwork of drainage canals around the outer edge of the iris (the colored part of the eye). Think of it as a sink with the faucet turned on. The tissues that produce the fluid are the faucets, and for the sink not to overflow, the draining canals of the eye (like the drain pipes connected to the sink) must remain open and unobstructed.

The internal pressure in the eye depends on how much fluid it contains and whether the fluid can pass freely in and out. As we grow older, the drainage canals begin to operate more slowly. They also angle and bend, interfering with this flow. As a result, fluid backs up and stagnates within the eye, raising its pressure. This condition, called *primary open-angle glaucoma*, accounts for at least 60 percent of glaucoma in the elderly. It is an insidious process that rarely causes any symptoms until the optic nerve is damaged and vision is lost. Once that happens, sight cannot be restored, so prevention and early treatment are key. *Increased pressure in the eye results in glaucoma only if has been undetected and left untreated for any length of time.*

The more serious but much less common form of glaucoma is *acute angle-closure glaucoma*. Instead of a slow, progressive buildup of fluid pressure within the eye, the canals suddenly become obstructed. This results in various acute symptoms, including loss of vision, pain in the eyes, headache, nausea and vomiting, and the appearance of rainbow halos when you look at lights. *This is a medical emergency.* Unless it is treated quickly, blindness can occur within hours.

Fortunately, glaucoma is easy to diagnose and treat. It requires only regular examinations after age 35 by an ophthalmologist. If you're found to have elevated intraocular pressure, it can be normalized with several kinds of eyedrops. The most widely used are the beta-blockers, an example of which is Timoptic (timolol). They lower eye pressure by decreasing production of aqueous humor.

Beta-blockers also are used orally and by injection for other purposes—to treat heart failure, high blood pressure, and certain cardiac rhythm disorders. They're called beta-blockers because they block the production of adrenaline-like substances that help maintain a normal heart rate and prevent the bronchial tubes from going into spasm. Someone taking a beta-blocker is likely to have a slower heart rate and, if he or she has some underlying pulmonary problem, can develop wheezing and respiratory difficulties. Beta-blockers also can interact adversely with other cardiac drugs such as calcium channel blockers and digitalis.

What does this have to do with treating glaucoma? Any time a medication is introduced into the eye, some of it is absorbed through the tear ducts and enters the body's circulation. When prescribing a beta-blocker for a heart patient, doctors are careful to make sure that the drug is safe for the specific patient. However, the patient's vulnerability to the drug's adverse effects is not always taken into account when the drug is prescribed as an eyedrop, because such a seemingly small amount of drug is used. The problem is further compounded by the fact that many people have respiratory problems of which they are unaware or that are not obvious, especially to an eye doctor. In such cases, beta-blocker eyedrops can have serious consequences similar to those caused by their orally administered counterparts.

■ HERE'S WHAT'S NEW

Researchers at the Institute of Ophthalmology in London compared the findings in 2,600 glaucoma patients being treated with beta-blocker eyedrops with 9,000 people who had normal eye pressure. Those taking the drops, many of whom had no known history of lung problems, had a greater incidence (1 in every 55) of respiratory symptoms that required medical attention than those who did not receive a beta-blocker.

■ THE BOTTOM LINE

These observations, which affect hundreds of thousands of people being treated for glaucoma, are significant. Although beta-blockers are among the most widely used drops to lower intraocular pressure, some people clearly should not take them.

Before you start one of these drugs, I strongly suggest that you have a spirometry (breathing) test. Most eye specialists don't routinely perform it, so you'll have to ask your general practitioner or internist to arrange it. A normal spirometry reading is fairly good evidence that you're a good candidate for beta-blocker eye drops—as far as your lungs are concerned. However, don't forget about your heart. Ask your internist if any of your other medications may interact with a beta-blocker. Also, if you've been told you have a slow heart rate, make sure it's monitored after you start the beta-blocker. Remember too that lung problems can develop at any time as you get older, so it's a good idea to have your lung function and your pulse rate checked periodically while you're taking the drug.

If for some reason you aren't a good candidate for beta-blocker therapy for your glaucoma (because you have lung disease or your heart rate is too slow), other treatment options are available. These include carbonic anhydrase inhibitors, prostaglandin analogs, alpha-2 agonists, and cholinergic drugs. Discuss them with your eye doctor.

If the increased pressure within the eye cannot be reduced with medication, several surgical laser procedures are available.

GASTROESOPHAGEAL REFLUX DISEASE (GERD)

The Heartburn-Sleep Connection

MILLIONS OF AMERICANS—as many as 20 percent of the population—suffer from the reflux of stomach acid into the food pipe. When the muscle in your lower esophagus is weak and doesn't close properly, acid, food, and liquid spill up from the stomach and into the food pipe. Doctors call this gastroesophageal reflux disease (GERD). Signs and symptoms include heartburn, choking, chest pain, and burping, all of which usually become worse when you lie down after a meal. You can control these symptoms with antacids, medications that reduce stomach acid production, and various maneuvers such as elevating the head of your bed to reduce the amount of acid reflux when you lie down.

I'm amazed at how often a problem in one system of the body can affect other seemingly unrelated functions. For example, someone with premature heart disease may have a horizontal crease in each ear lobe. Or someone with jaundice due to liver disease or gall-bladder duct obstruction may itch all over. Here are some other examples.

Researchers found that among a group of 330 patients with obstructive sleep apnea—a condition of disturbed sleep patterns during which breathing stops for as long as 10 seconds, is followed by a gasp, and then resumes once more—62 percent of them also had GERD.

Patients with obstructive sleep apnea usually are treated with continuous positive airway pressure (CPAP). They are fitted with a mask attached to a machine that delivers pressurized air (not oxygen) through the nostrils. This keeps the airways open and prevents the breathing interruptions.

■ HERE'S WHAT'S NEW

Recent studies have shown that almost half the patients with sleep apnea who also have GERD experience improvement in their gastric reflux symptoms when treated with CPAP. That shouldn't come as a surprise. By increasing pressure in the chest, CPAP prevents acid from backing up into the esophagus.

And the simplest news yet: Chewing gum can also provide some temporary relief of GERD symptoms. According to researchers at Kings College in London, it does so first by stimulating swallowing that in turn helps clear acid from the food pipe. Second, and perhaps more important, it also increases secretion of saliva. The alkaline saliva neutralizes some of the excess acid in the upper gastrointestinal tract.

■ THE BOTTOM LINE

If you have both GERD and sleep apnea, and conventional therapy has not provided enough relief of your indigestion symptoms, try CPAP during the night.

In addition to everything else you do for your GERD, chew some gum, even though Medicare probably won't reimburse you for it.

When GERD Is Really Bad

As MENTIONED, standard treatments for gastroesophageal reflux disease include taking antacids and other medications such as H$_2$ blockers Prevacid (lansoprazole) and Nexium (esomeprazole) to reduce acid production by the stomach, and keeping the bed or the upper body elevated when lying down after eating. Continuous positive airway pressure (CPAP), which is normally used to treat sleep apnea, can also reduce the severity of GERD by increasing the pressure in the chest.

■ HERE'S WHAT'S NEW

Researchers have recently developed a special liquid polymer (a chemical found in myriad products ranging from hair spray to plastic) that can be injected into the lower esophagus. It strengthens the muscle fibers so they stay shut and prevent reflux.

The manufacturers of this drug (marketed under the brand name Enteryx) reported to the FDA that it effectively reduces symptoms of GERD, at least over the short term. Patients treated with it required fewer antacids and similar drugs. One year after receiving the injection, two-thirds of patients were able to get along without any medication. Enteryx apparently has no major adverse effects (at least in the first year), though some patients did complain of irritation of the esophagus for months after the injection. The FDA has approved Enteryx for use in the United States.

■ THE BOTTOM LINE

GERD usually can be adequately controlled by well-tolerated oral medications. However, the few people who do not respond to conventional therapy should try CPAP. When symptoms are severe and persistent, ask your doctor about Enteryx. When it's injected into the lower esophageal muscle, it may strengthen the muscle sufficiently to reduce the upward leak of acid.

HEART DISEASE

New Treatments for Weak Hearts

THE MAIN FUNCTION OF THE HEART is to pump oxygen-rich blood to every part of the body—around the clock, every day of the year, for as long as you live. However, several conditions can weaken the force with which it does so, including a previous heart attack; long-standing untreated high blood pressure (against which the heart has been pumping to get its blood into the arteries); disease that has damaged one or more of the four heart valves; a disease of the heart muscle itself (cardiomyopathy); infections, mostly viral; and other conditions that involve and damage the heart muscle.

When cardiac function is compromised for any reason, the heart tries to maintain its ability to expel the necessary amounts of blood by enlarging and becoming thicker. When it can no longer do so, it "gives up," dilates, and weakens. In other words, it "fails" and the patient is then said to have congestive heart failure. The amount of blood delivered to the rest of the body decreases and backs up into the lungs. As a result, the lungs become congested and the patient is short of breath. The feet also swell because when the lungs are congested, blood backs up into the veins, and down the legs.

The first approach to treating heart failure is to remove any ongoing condition that is causing or perpetuating it. For example, if you have high blood pressure, keep it under control. Try to normalize high C-reactive protein and homocysteine levels (see pages 124 and 127). If you're diabetic, recent research has shown that you can lower your chances of developing heart failure by using a combination of statin drugs, angiotensin-converting enzyme (ACE) inhibitors, and beta-blockers. If you've had a heart attack that has already knocked out some muscle, angioplasty or bypass surgery can open any other vessels that are ready to close up, thus preventing another heart attack. If a diseased, malformed valve is placing a burden on your heart, it should be repaired or replaced.

Other specific treatments are available, ranging from drug therapy to heart transplants. Until fairly recently, the three most important and widely used drugs for this purpose were digitalis, diuretics (to eliminate any retained fluid), and ACE inhibitors, whose prototype is Capoten (captopril). Although they remain effective and continue to be prescribed for most patients with heart failure, several other drugs have become available that can further prolong survival and improve the quality of life.

■ HERE'S WHAT'S NEW

Drugs. For many years after their discovery, beta-blockers were used mainly to lower blood pressure, slow a rapidly beating heart, correct rhythm abnormalities, and relieve angina (chest pain). Doctors were told specifically to avoid prescribing them for patients with heart failure, in the mistaken belief that they further weaken the heart muscle. But recent research has confirmed their usefulness in this condition.

There are several different beta-blockers and, for practical purposes, one is as good as another. However, several studies have shown that one in particular, Coreg (carvedilol) may be more effective than the others in treating heart failure. Equally impressive was the observation that children with severe congestive heart failure who were placed on a heart transplant waiting list sometimes could be removed from that list because they improved so much with the drug. (Coreg's greater effectiveness than other beta-blockers is limited to heart failure therapy and does not necessarily apply to other situations, such as reducing heart rate, relieving angina, and controlling rhythm disorders.)

Beta-blockers are now also routinely prescribed after a heart attack, even in the absence of congestive failure. However, they can aggravate other disorders such as chronic lung disease and arterial disease in the legs that causes pain on walking. Although beta-blockers, in conjunction with ACE inhibitors and statins, are beneficial for diabetics, they can mask the symptoms of a low blood glucose level.

Continuous positive airway pressure (CPAP). Obstructive sleep apnea—disturbed sleep patterns during which breathing stops for as long as 10 seconds—is commonly associated with coronary artery disease and high blood pressure. About 30 percent of patients with congestive heart failure also have obstructive sleep apnea.

Continuous positive airway pressure keeps airways open and prevents the breathing interruptions in people with sleep apnea. Patients are fitted with a mask attached to a machine that delivers pressurized air (not oxygen) through the nostrils.

CPAP also helps congestive heart failure that accompanies obstructive sleep apnea. Patients in whom CPAP was added to the standard heart failure treatment enjoyed better cardiac function as shown by a lower daytime systolic blood pressure (the top number), a slower heart rate, and improved pumping action of the heart.

Transplants. In addition to medication, some stunning new technological advances have emerged for severely weakened hearts. A heart transplant is the treatment of choice, but unfortunately there are not nearly enough hearts to go around. The lucky few who do receive them have a much better quality of life than those who were given them years ago, thanks to the new antirejection drugs available today. A 42-year-old woman who was given a human heart transplant in 1996 recently climbed the 14,000-foot Mount Matterhorn in Switzerland. (A few years before the transplant, her heart muscle had been severely damaged by a virus.)

Artificial hearts. For those who need a new heart but can't wait for a transplant, new types of "artificial" hearts, or more accurately "assist devices," enable them to enjoy an acceptable quality of life. The Jarvik heart is the prototype of several others that were approved this past year. The patient's own heart is left in place, but an assist device is placed inside the left ventricle (the main chamber of the heart that does most of the pumping). It boosts the ability of the heart muscle to contract so that it can provide enough blood with each beat.

These devices were originally designed as temporary solutions for those waiting for heart transplants. However, they are functioning so well that, in many cases, heart transplants are not required. I know one such patient with an implanted Jarvik heart who says he feels better than he did before he developed heart trouble and who for the past 3 years has been hiking. (Before his surgery, he was unable to walk to the next room!)

The main problems with assist devices, besides the possibility of mechanical failure, are infection and bleeding. But these are becoming less frequent. Their track record? Some 52 percent of patients with end-stage heart failure survive for 1 year after implantation, as compared with only 25 percent treated with drug therapy. Remember, however, that these are the sickest of the sick. At 2 years, only 8 percent undergoing medical treatment alone survive, compared to nearly 25 percent of those with left ventricular assist devices. As researchers continue to solve these technical problems, the units will be more widely used.

The totally implanted heart also is being improved. Here, the patient's own heart is actually removed and replaced with an implanted device the size of a fist. Although some patients have survived a relatively short time, these hearts have not yet achieved the kind of results that should inspire you to rush to get one.

Other implant devices. Many patients with weak hearts are vulnerable to sudden death due to a rhythm disorder of the left ventricle. Most cardiologists are now convinced that these patients should receive an implantable defibrillator. This device just sits there until a life-threatening arrhythmia develops, at which point it kicks in and terminates the abnormal rhythm by shocking the heart. If everyone eligible for such a defibrillator were to receive one, there could be 200,000 fewer sudden deaths in the United States alone.

When the heart is weak, the left and right ventricles do not beat simultaneously, which reduces their efficiency. For such patients who have a specific kind of abnormality on their electrocardiogram, a "synchronizing" pacemaker can, along with the defibrillator, improve symptoms and prolong life. This pacemaker stimulates both ventricles so they contract together, thus improving the cardiac output. Ask your cardiologist whether you are a candidate for such a synchronizing device.

■ THE BOTTOM LINE

The best way to deal with heart failure is to prevent it. However, a host of drugs is now available, the beta-blockers among them, that can greatly improve the duration and quality of life in patients with weak hearts. In addition, defibrillators, "synchronizing" pacemakers, and artificial heart assists have reduced the need for difficult-to-get heart transplants and have prolonged the lives of many people.

Surviving Cardiac Arrest

EVERY YEAR, more than 220,000 Americans suddenly collapse and die from cardiac arrest. In many cases, there's no warning. They're alive one moment and dead the next. The heart suddenly stops pumping blood; the brain (and the rest of the body) receives no nourishment and so stops functioning. Unless the arrest is treated and normal heart action restored within 4 to 6 minutes, the person dies. This lethal rhythm is not necessarily a result of weakness of the heart muscle (although arrest often occurs in people with heart failure) but instead is a disorder of the cardiac electrical system. Most patients who suffer cardiac arrest have some type of underlying heart disease, whether or not they are aware of it.

Cardiac arrest occurs in two ways. In about 25 percent of cases, the heart either slows down dramatically, beating only a few times a minute instead of the normal 60 to 80 beats per minute, or stops. In the remaining 75 percent of cases, ventricular fibrillation causes the arrest. In these cases, instead of contracting and expelling blood, the ventricles quiver ineffectively like a bag of worms and do not expel any blood.

The most effective way to deal with cardiac arrest is shock—delivered by a pacemaker to get the heart beating again if it has stopped or a defibrillator to jolt it back to normal rhythm. These machines originally were designed for use in ambulances and wherever people congregated in large numbers—airplanes, stadiums, casinos, large corporate offices, amusement parks. Personnel working in those areas were taught how to use them. It's not clear how many lives public defibrillators have actually saved. Part of the problem with the machines is that they require the immediate presence of someone who knows when and how to use them.

The next step in the defibrillator saga was the invention of a tiny machine that is implanted in the heart of a vulnerable person to sense life-threatening rhythm and shock it back to normal. These devices have saved thousands of lives. I have patients with such internal defibrillators who lead an otherwise normal existence except that from time to time they are spontaneously shocked out of rhythm abnormalities that would otherwise kill them.

■ HERE'S WHAT'S NEW

The latest advance in this area is the development and FDA approval of home defibrillators. Because 70 percent of cardiac arrests occur at home, this will have a great impact on the threat of sudden death. Although no one is immune to this catastrophe, most victims are men in their sixties with a history of heart disease. The main users of the home defibrillators are their wives.

The home defibrillator requires a doctor's prescription and costs between $2,000 and $2,500. The machine is user-friendly. It's programmed to determine whether a person actually needs the shock. So if a family member turns on the machine but the condition is, say, a stroke and not cardiac arrest, the machine will not go into the shock mode. The unit is battery-operated and beeps when the battery is low.

Although I recommend these units to selected patients who are at risk for cardiac arrest, the American Heart Association does not yet endorse their universal use. It wants more evidence that it will save lives. The National Institutes of Health has initiated a study of 7,000 people at high risk. Family members of half the subjects will be trained in CPR; families of the other half will be given defibrillators. At the end of 4 years, the results for both groups will be tallied. In the meantime, the FDA has ordered the manufacturers to keep track of the results that are reported to them.

■ THE BOTTOM LINE

Home defibrillators are not for healthy people. Who wants to come home from a hard day's work and see one of these units next to the dining room table or the bed? But if you have coronary artery disease or are taking medication for an arrhythmia, ask your doctor if you are a candidate for cardiac arrest, no matter how remote the possibility. If you are and you don't live alone, I suggest you invest in a home defibrillator. You may also want to consider it if you need one implanted but are too sick to have the procedure done.

The ABCs of C-RP

DURING THIS PAST YEAR, there has been renewed interest in the C-reactive protein (C-RP) blood test, a diagnostic tool that has been around for 65 years. Since this protein is elevated in the presence of obvious inflammation due to any cause, the C-RP test was used to diagnose and monitor the progress of infections and certain diseases that affect the immune system, such as rheumatoid arthritis. Recently, we have become aware that various parts of the body can be inflamed without causing any symptoms—no fever, no pain, no symptoms whatsoever. This silent process may indicate the presence of a life-threatening condition when it involves the lining of a blood vessel in the heart or brain. Such inflammation usually doesn't cause symptoms, but it leaves the blood vessel prone to clogging and obstructing the flow of blood within it.

Such inflammation, albeit silent, has been found to be as important a risk factor for heart disease as are conventionally recognized ones. The clogging occurs because when any plaques already present in these inflamed vessels rupture, the resulting debris obstructs the vessels and causes a heart attack or stroke. Silent inflammation explains why some people who have no other apparent risk factors for vascular disease and who are seemingly in good health nevertheless develop heart attacks or strokes in the prime of their lives. C-RP not only is an indicator of underlying inflammation but also is believed to stimulate the release of inflammatory substances called cytokines that further promote clotting in the arteries.

■ HERE'S WHAT'S NEW

C-reactive protein is now considered a better predictor of vulnerability to arteriosclerosis and its consequences than is a high LDL (bad cholesterol) level. Because a person with a high C-RP level is at twice the risk of having a heart attack or stroke, regardless of cholesterol level, knowing your C-RP level is important. It can easily be determined by a blood test that costs around $15 to $20. The average reading in this country is 1.5; levels of 3 or higher are an important warning for you to take whatever steps are necessary to protect yourself.

What should you do about a high C-RP level? Will lowering it reduce your risk of vascular disease? Most doctors think so, but this has not yet been proven. A large trial of 15,000 people that began in January 2003 may provide the answer. Until then, here's what I suggest.

Rule out an infection somewhere in the body. Your doctor should make sure that you don't have an underlying infection or an autoimmune disease, such as rheumatoid arthritis or lupus, that could account for the high C-RP level.

Focus on the vascular system. You should have an electrocardiogram, a stress test, and a sonogram of the carotid arteries in the neck to look for evidence of arteriosclerosis. I also sometimes order an ultrafast CT scan of the chest or an equivalent test to identify calcium deposits in and around the coronary arteries.

Control your risk factors. If your C-RP level is high, control any other risk factors you may have. However, even if you have none, check your blood pressure; follow a diet low in saturated fat and rich in oily fish; eat lots of fruit, vegetables, and whole grains; exercise regularly; try to achieve ideal weight; and if you smoke, quit.

Consider taking a statin drug. The following is a key recommendation, regardless of your cholesterol level. Besides normalizing blood fats, statin drugs such as Lipitor (atorvastatin) and Pravachol (pravastatin) also reduce inflammation, thus stabilizing any plaques in your coronary arteries and reducing the likelihood of their clotting. They have been shown to lower C-RP by 15 to 25 percent. A recent study shows that high doses of statin drugs (80 milligrams of Lipitor) decreased C-RP levels by almost 30 percent in patients with type 2 diabetes (who are especially vulnerable to vascular disease).

Take a drink. Adults who drank three to four glasses of beer with dinner lowered their C-RP levels by about 35 percent after 3 weeks, presumably because of the anti-inflammatory properties of alcohol. As far as I'm concerned, that's a lot of beer, with or without dinner! My advice is to have a cocktail or a glass or two of wine with your evening meal—but no more than that. More is not better, especially if you'll be driving later on.

Get help from a pill. In another study, people who took a multivitamin also dropped their C-RP levels (and lowered their homocysteine levels as well—see page 128). The researchers in this particular study believe that this beneficial effect was a result of vitamins B and C. (Several other studies have found no benefit from multivitamins overall.) The antibiotic Vibramycin (doxycycline), widely used to treat gum disease, was recently found to lower C-RP levels by nearly 50 percent in patients with acute heart attacks. A daily aspirin or other nonsteroidal anti-inflammatory drug (taken after meals) also should be standard therapy for a high C-RP level.

■ THE BOTTOM LINE

Make sure the C-RP test is part of your routine physical. If your level is elevated, start immediately to control your risk factors and ask your doctor about taking a statin drug, regardless of your cholesterol level and especially if you're diabetic.

If your cholesterol level is normal or low, should you have a C-RP test anyway? You bet! Although the American Heart Association and the Centers for Disease Control and Prevention recommend routine C-RP testing only for people at risk of heart disease, in my own practice I do it for virtually every adult patient. Many people have heart attacks and strokes even with no risk factors other than high C-RP levels.

What if your cholesterol level is high and you know you're already at increased risk for vascular disease? Should you have the C-RP test anyway? I believe it's a good idea because if both cholesterol and C-RP levels are high, you are at substantially greater risk and should be more aggressive about preventive measures.

How (And Why) to Lower Your Homocysteine

HOMOCYSTEINE is a protein by-product of normal metabolism. Its levels can be measured in the blood. When they're too high, you're at increased risk for a heart attack, high blood pressure, stroke, and blood clots in the deep veins of the legs. The upper limit of normal depends on the laboratory performing the test but should be less than 15 micromol per liter.

■ HERE'S WHAT'S NEW

Besides the risks noted above, new evidence suggests that a high homocysteine blood level is also associated with sudden death, especially in diabetics, and twice the risk of Alzheimer's disease, regardless of age or sex.

In people who lack vitamin B, usually because they don't get enough in their diets, homocysteine levels rise. Recent research has shown that these elevations can be reduced by 25 to 35 percent with a combination of B vitamins—specifically folic acid and vitamins B_6 and B_{12}. These vitamins break down the homocysteine, thus preventing its accumulation. (Folic acid alone will lower homocysteine levels but not as much as when combined with the other two B vitamins.)

One study found that patients who took these supplements for 6 months after undergoing angioplasty were 32 percent less likely to suffer another blockage, have a heart attack, or die during the following year. The hard proof that lowering homocysteine actually prevents heart attacks is not yet in, but most researchers are confident that it will do so.

As with many health breakthroughs, these findings are not without debate. New research suggests that high doses of folic acid may trigger cell overgrowth in the coronary arteries and actually predispose the arteries to early closure after angioplasty. Because this has been observed only with high doses of folic acid, you should limit your intake of folic acid to 1 milligram a day.

■ THE BOTTOM LINE

If your homocysteine level is high, you should take 1 milligram of folic acid a day (current U.S. dietary recommendations call for only 0.4 milligram) as well as 10 milligrams of vitamin B_6 and 400 micrograms (0.4 milligram) of vitamin B_{12}. You should also have your homocysteine levels checked two or three times a year.

Eating foods rich in the B vitamins (leafy green vegetables, low-fat dairy products, citrus fruits and juices, whole wheat bread, cereals, and dry beans) is also useful, but getting the right amount in the diet is more difficult than taking a fixed, adequate dose in a pill every morning. So even if you decide to go the diet route, take a multivitamin containing folic acid every morning just to be sure.

Even Newer Tests

IT'S INTERESTING to look back at how our understanding of the risk factors of cardiovascular disease has evolved over the years. When I graduated from medical school, the only definite one was a family history of the disease. If either of your parents, one or more siblings, or any other immediate blood relatives had cardiovascular problems at an early age, you were considered vulnerable.

As we continue to learn more about how and why arteries become diseased and interfere with blood flow to various organs, we realize that there are several other indicators of vulnerability to premature heart disease and stroke. These include cigarette smoking, lack of regular physical exercise, overweight, diabetes, high blood pressure, and abnormal blood fat levels, including cholesterol levels. A person's risk profile is now largely based on an assessment of all these risk factors.

Every now and then, however, men and women who do not fit into any of these categories are affected with vascular disease at an early age. For example, between one-third and one-half of heart attacks occur in people with normal cholesterol levels. Doctors have been searching for ways to identify these patients so as to forestall their disease. Recently, we have begun to recognize the importance of silent inflammation of the blood vessels (when the blood vessel lining is inflamed and prone to clogging but causes no acute symptoms) as yet another marker and contributing factor to premature vascular disease. As mentioned earlier, the C-reactive protein test, a reflection of such inflammation, has now been shown to predict vulnerability to heart attack and stroke more accurately than even the much vaunted "bad" cholesterol (LDL). Doctors are now evaluating ways of reducing high C-RP readings in an attempt to reduce the risk of heart disease.

■ HERE'S WHAT'S NEW

Several large clinical trials have indicated that besides C-RP levels, another predictor of heart disease risk that is more accurate than LDL cholesterol concentration in the blood is the level of apolipoprotein (Apo for short) in the blood.

Apolipoproteins are tiny fat particles—of which there are several varieties (the best known are ApoA1 and ApoB)—that circulate in the blood. According to studies published in the medical journal *The Lancet*, a high ApoB level or a high ApoB:ApoA1 ratio is a very sensitive indicator of vulnerability to vascular disease. Researchers believe that doctors should now routinely measure these apolipoproteins, especially in at-risk patients. The term *apolipoprotein* sounds intimidating, but this test is actually easier to perform than a cholesterol screen and doesn't require the patient to fast beforehand.

Finally, the FDA has approved yet another test, this one specifically recommended for those with low or normal cholesterol levels who are considered at risk for vascular disease because of other risk factors. Called the PLAC test, it measures an enzyme known as PLA2 that is active in the inflammatory process of the lining of the small arteries. Patients with high concentrations of this enzyme have twice the risk of heart attacks, despite low levels of LDL cholesterol. The cost of this latest test is about $16, which is about the same as the C-RP analysis.

■ THE BOTTOM LINE

New evidence suggests that every routine checkup of adult males and females should include tests for vulnerability to premature heart disease. This evaluation should consist of a careful family history, complete physical examination, electrocardiogram at rest and/or after exercise, and blood analyses for levels of total cholesterol, LDL, HDL, homocysteine, blood glucose, and C-RP. It now appears that looking at ApoB (ideally, the ApoB:ApoA1 ratio) as well as the PLAC test can provide even greater predictability of premature heart disease.

WHAT THE DOCTOR ORDERED?

THE FISH OIL DEBATE ■ Several studies over the years have suggested that eating fish, especially oily ones, reduces the risk of heart attack. The omega-3 fatty acids that fish contain help lower blood pressure a little, reduce levels of other harmful fats, inhibit the growth of artery-blocking plaques, prevent the formation of arterial blood clots, and decrease the incidence of heart disease in diabetics. In addition to protecting the heart, omega-3s are also good for the eyes and reduce airway constriction spasm in asthmatics as well.

During the past year several conflicting reports have emerged about how much fish one should eat. Some also emphasize the potential danger of the mercury content in certain fish; others are less concerned. Unless you read *all* these studies, you may not get a balanced view of what is good for you—and what may be bad.

HERE'S WHAT'S NEW

Originally, the American Heart Association (AHA) recommended two servings a week of oily fish, both for healthy individuals and for people with heart disease. They then revised this advice because several large clinical trials found that individuals with heart disease need more than two servings. The AHA now recommends eating fish such as mackerel, lake trout, herring, sardines, tuna, and salmon *every day* to get the required 1 gram of the necessary omega-3 fatty acids. You may need even more if your blood triglyceride levels are elevated. (But then tell your doctor how much you're eating, because eating too much fish may interfere with the clotting mechanism of the blood and cause excessive bleeding.)

The AHA recommends that healthy people continue to eat two servings of oily fish a week. Pregnant women, nursing mothers, and children should avoid mackerel, tilefish, swordfish, tuna, and shark. These fish contain high levels of mercury, dioxins, and PCBs, chemicals that are potentially hazardous to children's nervous systems. However, cooked shellfish, canned fish, and smaller ocean fish are safe. The latest blockbuster news about eating most types of fish during pregnancy is that the mercury levels in most fish do not affect the fetus in any way, least of all neurologically. However, researchers still caution that the above-mentioned varieties containing the highest amounts of mercury should probably be avoided.

So far, so good. But hot on the heels of the AHA advice there appeared two conflicting reports in the *New England Journal of Medicine*. One stated that mercury levels in men who'd had heart attacks were 15 percent higher than levels in healthy men. Researchers believe that the toxic effects of mercury in fish not only cancel out the cardiovascular benefits of the omega-3 fatty acids but actually make matters worse. However, not everyone agrees. A second study in the same journal found that there was no correlation between eating fish, mercury levels, and heart attacks. What's a consumer to think?

Meanwhile, studies continue to find even more benefits from fish. One report in the *Journal of the American Medical Association* concluded that men who consumed 3 to 5 ounces of fish only one to three times a month were 43 percent less likely to have a stroke during the next 12 years!

There appears to be yet another important reason to eat lots of oily fish like salmon, tuna, and bluefish—at least twice a week. The fatty acids they contain prevent life-threatening cardiac arrhythmias. These fatty acids, which are stored in the cell membranes of the heart, control the entry and exit of chemicals such as calcium that can predispose the heart to dangerous rhythm disturbances. The researchers are so impressed with the protective action of the fatty acids against sudden death that they are recommending that people take omega-3 supplements, because the necessary 1 gram a day may not be available through diet alone.

Another study, reported in the British Medical Journal, looked at the effects of regular intake of fish in more than 1,600 people older than age 68 living in southwest France. Researchers found that those who ate fish regularly for at least 7 years had a substantially lower incidence of Alzheimer's disease. Anyone who had eaten fish at least once a week derived some benefit, but the more fish they consumed, the better off they were.

But wait! It isn't as simple as that. Just eating fish is not enough. How you prepare it is also important, according to a study reported in the journal Circulation. Baking or broiling is the way to go. In a large, population-based study of adults older than 65, fried fish and fish sandwiches offered no beneficial cardiac effects.

THE BOTTOM LINE

Eating fish is clearly good for you. Despite all the warnings about mercury, I still believe that if you have heart disease, the more fish you eat—especially oily ones such as salmon and tuna—the better. And if you don't like fish or can't afford it, buy omega-3 supplements to make sure you consume at least 1 gram a day. Omega Brite, Solgar, and TwinLabs are reliable brands. Unless properly made, the oil can become rancid.

> Pregnant women should limit consumption only of ocean-going fish that contain the highest concentrations of mercury, including mackerel, tilefish, swordfish, tuna, and shark, although canned fish is safe.
>
> Finally, whatever fish you end up eating, make sure you don't fry it! ▪

Mammograms to Detect Heart Disease

THIS YEAR one of the most hallowed medical theories refuted by new research findings was that menopausal women should take hormone replacement therapy (HRT). It not only fails to protect against vascular diseases but also may increase the risk (see page 181).

The value and cost-effectiveness of another time-honored practice, the regular mammogram, was also for a time questioned (see page 44). After much debate, the consensus appears to be that, properly interpreted (something you shouldn't take for granted, because diagnostic skills vary greatly among radiologists), mammograms are useful and every woman should have one regularly starting just before menopause or soon after (that is, between ages 40 and 50).

▪ HERE'S WHAT'S NEW

Besides finding cancer in the breast before a woman or her doctor can feel it, mammograms can also indicate the presence of heart disease early in the game. That's because the x-rays beamed at the breasts also can identify calcifications in the coronary arteries. Women with these calcifications are 20 percent more likely to develop heart disease.

▪ THE BOTTOM LINE

Do not have a mammogram just to look for evidence of heart disease. However, when the radiologist reports the findings to you, ask whether he or she happened to see any calcifications in your coronary arteries. If they were present (and that's more likely in women older than age 60), let your doctor know. You may then be advised to undergo other tests to clarify their significance because, according to researchers at the Mayo Clinic, there's a one in five chance that coronary calcifications detected this way reflect underlying heart disease.

When to Say No to Antioxidants

THERE IS WIDESPREAD BELIEF that antioxidants prevent heart disease, reduce its severity, or both. The most popular antioxidants in the United States are vitamins C and E and beta-carotene.

▪ HERE'S WHAT'S NEW

Recent research indicates that most adult diabetics should take a cholesterol-lowering drug, such as a statin, even if their cholesterol levels are normal and they don't have heart disease. These medications were originally recommended only for people with high cholesterol levels. However, in a new study of 20,000 diabetics, those taking a 40-milligram tablet of Zocor (simvastatin)—one of several available statins—had a 25 percent lower risk of subsequent cardiovascular events such as a heart attack.

New findings by researchers at the University of Washington may surprise you. The scientists evaluated 160 people with heart disease who were taking cholesterol-lowering drugs (Zocor and niacin). Half of the patients were also taking one or more antioxidants. After 3 years, the incidence of new vascular disease—including death, stroke, another heart attack, or the need for angioplasty or bypass surgery—was much lower (3 percent) among those who took the anticholesterol medication *without* the antioxidants. The subjects receiving both antioxidants *and* cholesterol-lowering drugs experienced a 14 percent incidence of these events—almost four times as many as the others.

In a British study of 20,000 patients taking antioxidants alone (that is, without cholesterol-lowering drugs), the antioxidants had no effect whatsoever on the incidence of vascular disease.

Now here's the clincher. In the most recent evaluation of the effectiveness of antioxidants on the cardiovascular system, researchers at the Cleveland Clinic Foundation analyzed the results from 15 studies involving 220,000 people, most of whom were either especially vulnerable to heart and vascular disease or already had it. All of them had been followed for as long as 12 years, enough time to tell whether something works or doesn't. The study found that vitamin E and beta-carotene, alone or together, did not improve a person's vascular status. In fact, beta-carotene alone actually *increased* the risk of cardiovascular disease as well as death from any cause.

Staunch believers in these vitamins are now suggesting that they help prevent vascular disease in *healthy* people, but not in those already affected. That's an interesting possibility, and only time and further studies will yield the answer. As for me personally, I have stopped taking antioxidant supplements but I continue to consume these nutrients by eating foods in which they are plentiful. That means at least five servings of fresh fruits and vegetables every day.

■ THE BOTTOM LINE

Most people with heart disease who take a cholesterol-lowering drug should avoid antioxidant supplements. Though antioxidants reduce the incidence of upper-respiratory tract infections in people with diabetes, diabetics on a cholesterol-lowering drug should not take these supplements, especially if they already have some evidence of vascular disease. It's better to have a cold than a heart attack!

However, if you are at risk for colon cancer because of a strong family history, and you are also a nonsmoker and nondrinker, the antioxidant beta-carotene may decrease your chances of developing this malignancy (see page 79).

Drink Wisely—Or Not at All

WE'VE KNOWN FOR SEVERAL YEARS that alcohol in moderation protects men and post-menopausal women against heart disease. It probably does so by raising blood levels of HDL (the "good" cholesterol) and certain cardioprotective enzymes and proteins. Every now and then you'll read that a particular form of alcohol is more effective than others—be it beer, white wine, or red wine—the latter presumably because of the resveratrol content found in the skin of grapes. (Resveratrol is a chemical with many different properties, but it's best known as an antioxidant.)

■ HERE'S WHAT'S NEW

The latest studies relating to alcohol's effect on the heart emphasize that it isn't the kind of alcohol you drink or whether you take it with a meal that's important. The key appears to be *how much* and *how often* you imbibe.

In a 12-year study of 38,000 male health professionals ages 40 to 75, none of whom had heart disease, researchers found that those who consumed any type of alcoholic beverage 3 or more days a week reduced their risk of heart attack by about one-third, as compared with those who drank less alcohol. Two drinks a day appeared to be the optimal amount; more was not better.

■ THE BOTTOM LINE

If you enjoy moderate social drinking, continue to do so. But don't ignore other risk factors, including weight, smoking, cholesterol levels, and exercise. Most important, don't interpret this new information as a prescription to start drinking if you've never done so before, because despite these findings, alcohol can hurt more than it helps. As one editorial in the *New England Journal of Medicine* put it, if alcohol were a new drug, the FDA would probably not approve it. Its many toxic effects and complications—the risk of addiction; the violence and accidents that occur with its use; the damage to the liver, gastrointestinal tract, brain, kidneys, and even the heart in some cases—far outweigh its benefits. There are other, more effective and less risky ways to reduce your risk of heart disease.

Angioplasty and the New Stents

IT WASN'T LONG AGO that the only way for doctors to get blood flowing through a clogged coronary artery was to perform a bypass operation. Many thousands of these surgeries were done throughout the country, with excellent results. They are still being performed, but much less frequently. That's because angioplasty, the art of ballooning open these blood vessels, has been so successfully refined. In my own practice, for every patient I refer for a bypass operation, I send 10 for angioplasty.

Angioplasty has become even more successful since the development of stents, little mesh "sleeves" that are placed inside the artery to keep them open after blood flow has been restored. These stents have further reduced the chances of clots reforming after the angioplasty balloon compresses the obstructing plaques against the artery wall.

■ HERE'S WHAT'S NEW

Although stenting has reduced the incidence of reclosure after ballooning, the incidence has nevertheless remained at about 30 percent, especially in smaller coronary arteries in which blood flow is not as brisk.

In April 2003, a new stent was released that has lowered the incidence of closure to less than 10 percent. It is coated with the drug rapamycin. When applied to the stents, rapamycin prevents those changes in the wall of the artery that ultimately lead to clot formation. This new technology will further reduce the need for coronary bypass surgery.

■ THE BOTTOM LINE

If you have angina or other symptoms of coronary artery narrowing, an angiogram will determine the extent and location of the blockage. In many cases, these arteries can be ballooned open with angioplasty and then stented. Ideally, you should have a rapamycin-coated stent. Unfortunately, because of its higher cost, this stent is not always made available. I am told that some insurance carriers will pay for it only after the older devices have failed. If you have any say in the matter, insist on a rapamycin-coated stent to keep your ballooned artery open.

The Latest Aspirin News

IT'S A RARE MEDICAL MEETING where some researcher fails to come up with yet another benefit of aspirin for a malady (heart disease, cancer, pain—you name it). What started as a simple over-the-counter pill to reduce fever and control mild pain has evolved into what is arguably the most versatile drug available to mankind. It not only reduces elevated temperature and eases soreness but also helps prevent strokes, heart attacks, and various cancers. And that's probably only the beginning of the aspirin saga.

With regard to aspirin's role in vascular disease, we have known for years that it protects men who are at high risk for developing vascular problems (this is called primary prevention). An aspirin a day also reduces the risk of a second heart attack or stroke in men who've already had one (secondary prevention). Aspirin also interferes with blood clotting by acting on blood platelets so they don't clump together and form clots in the arteries. This is why someone taking aspirin for any reason bleeds more easily and why this drug is usually discontinued before an operation.

▪ HERE'S WHAT'S NEW

Aspirin is not just for men. Researchers always assumed, but never proved, that women also can benefit from aspirin. Now, scientists at Miami's Mount Sinai Medical Center and Heart Institute have found that aspirin does reduce the risk of a first heart attack in high-risk individuals of both sexes. Their conclusion is based on an analysis of results from five different studies. Some 55,000 subjects, 11,000 of them women, were divided into two groups—those who took daily aspirin (anywhere from 81 to 325 milligrams) and those who didn't. The aspirin protected both women and men, providing an overall reduction of 32 percent in the rate of heart attacks, strokes, and other vascular events.

High cholesterol level reduces aspirin's benefit. And here's a new twist. Recent research from the University of Maryland suggests that for aspirin to exert its protective effect on the cardiovascular system, the cholesterol level must be normal. When it's elevated, aspirin does not as efficiently prevent blood platelets from clumping and forming clots.

Low-dose and coated tablets aren't as effective. Two new studies have appeared, one of which, if true, will disappoint many users of aspirin, including me. Doctors running the stroke program at Northwestern Memorial Hospital in Chicago are suggesting that low-dose aspirin (81 milligrams), the so-called children's aspirin, is not nearly as effective in preventing the abnormal blood clotting that leads to heart attack and stroke as are higher strengths. Neither are the coated tablets.

The researchers observed that more than half of the 250 subjects who were taking aspirin experienced no anticlotting benefits and developed heart attacks and strokes. It turns out that they were taking either low-dose aspirin or coated tablets. For example, platelets were affected in only 44 percent of those taking the 81-milligram dose of aspirin, as compared with 72 percent of those on the 325-milligram dose. That's a big difference. As far as coating was concerned, it had no impact on platelets in 65 percent of cases, whereas the uncoated pills reduced clotting in 75 percent.

Aspirin shouldn't be combined with ibuprofen. Researchers in the United Kingdom found that combining aspirin with ibuprofen (such as Motrin) on a regular basis also interferes with its anticlotting properties. Many people, especially the elderly, use these two drugs together. They take aspirin for protection against vascular disease and ibuprofen or a similar drug to ease their aches and pains. In a well-conducted study, researchers found that those who took aspirin with ibuprofen on a regular basis were twice as likely to die of cardiovascular disease as people on aspirin alone.

■ THE BOTTOM LINE

Whether you're male or female, if you're at high risk for having a heart attack or stroke, take an aspirin every day and make sure your cholesterol level is within normal limits. If this advice were heeded, it's estimated that there would be 350,000 fewer heart attacks and other vascular events every year.

For the time being, until another study comes out refuting the above findings, you're better off taking the full-strength tablet (325 milligrams) of uncoated aspirin. However, if you are prone to stomach irritation or are a senior citizen, the larger dose may present a problem, so check with your doctor first.

WHAT THE DOCTOR ORDERED?

TAKE ASPIRIN, SPARE YOUR GUT

▓ Even the 81-milligram low-dose aspirin, including the enteric-coated form, can irritate your stomach and be more likely to cause gastrointestinal bleeding if you have a stomach ulcer.

HERE'S WHAT'S NEW

The latest research indicates that stomachache from aspirin may be due to something other than the drug—namely a bacterium called *Helicobacter pylori*. Researchers in Japan found that animals experimentally infected with *H. pylori* and given aspirin were much more likely to develop irritation of the stomach lining than those taking aspirin but free of *H. pylori*.

In humans, this bug often causes stomach ulcers (with and without aspirin on board) and has also been linked to gastric cancer.

Doctors at the Chinese University of Hong Kong who studied several hundred patients found that eliminating *H. pylori* with the appropriate antibiotics allowed them to take aspirin with few, if any, of the side effects they'd previously had (abdominal pain, gas, and indigestion).

THE BOTTOM LINE

If you must take aspirin regularly and find it irritates your stomach, or if you have a peptic ulcer, ask your doctor to check you for *H. pylori*. It's easy to do with either a breath test or a blood analysis. If you test positive, you can eradicate the organism by taking an antibiotic for 10 to 14 days. It's well worth it. Not only is there a good chance that you'll be able to take the aspirin you need but you may also reduce your risk of developing stomach cancer sometime in the future. And here's an extra bonus: If you have bad breath for which your dentist can find no cause, it just may come from your stomach—if any *H. pylori* is present. Getting rid of this bacterium may have you smelling very sweet, even when you exhale (see page 34).

It's also a good idea to be tested for *H. pylori* if you are taking a nonsteroidal anti-inflammatory drug such as ibuprofen to relieve chronic pain. If you are infected, eradicating the organism will minimize stomach irritation caused by these medications. However, you still may need to take an acid-reducing drug such as Prilosec (omeprazole) to further reduce your risk of bleeding. ■

HERPES

Don't Infect Your Newborn

THE HERPES SIMPLEX VIRUS (HSV) used to be a major concern for millions of Americans. However, the HIV/AIDS epidemic has taken center stage among the sexually transmitted diseases, and HSV is much less on our minds these days. What's more, the availability of new antiviral agents, such as Zovirax (acyclovir) and Famvir (famciclovir), has reduced both the recurrence rate of herpetic sores and the likelihood of transmission to an uninfected partner.

Although herpes is not as much of a threat as other sexually transmitted diseases such as human papillomavirus (which can lead to cervical cancer), it's still unpleasant and embarrassing. As the old Packard advertising slogan put it, just "ask the man (or woman) who owns one!"

Herpes may not be life threatening to an adult, but when a mother transmits the virus to her newborn, it can cause brain damage or even death. This is especially likely to happen if the woman recently acquired herpes, because her immune system has not yet had a chance to make antibodies to the virus, which she could pass to her child.

■ HERE'S WHAT'S NEW

It has long been suspected but never really proven that delivery by Cesarean section in women with active herpes significantly reduces the risk of infecting their newborns. Recent research has now shown this to be a fact. In a study of some 200 pregnant women who had herpes, only 1 percent of those who underwent Cesarean section gave birth to children with HSV, compared with the nearly 8 percent who delivered vaginally.

■ THE BOTTOM LINE

Obstetricians suggest that every pregnant woman be screened for genital herpes at her first prenatal care visit. If the test result is positive, she should be treated with one of the antiviral drugs mentioned above. If a woman was recently infected, she should consider having a Cesarean delivery, especially if she has genital sores.

It's also a good idea for the father to be checked, too. If the mother is negative but her partner is harboring the virus, he should take an antiviral drug at least during the entire pregnancy. He should always use a condom or abstain from sex until after the baby is born, in order not to infect the mother.

HIGH BLOOD PRESSURE

What Your Reading Really Means

CONSIDER THIS: Hypertension (high blood pressure) is a major killer and crippler in this country. More than 50 million Americans older than age 6 (this is not a typo—kids get it too) have high blood pressure. That's about one in every four of us. The incidence increases with age, so by age 75, two out of every three people are afflicted with it. Unfortunately, about one-third of those who have it don't know it. Among those who do, half are treated inadequately and continue to live with dangerously high blood pressure that ultimately weakens their hearts, clogs arteries throughout their bodies, and predisposes them to heart attacks, strokes, blindness, and kidney failure.

Despite this danger, there is little agreement among laypeople (and even doctors) about what constitutes high blood pressure. Ask around. You'll find some people who believe that a normal systolic pressure (the top number) is 100 plus your age. Others say the full reading should be 140/90. In terms of diastolic pressure (the lower figure), many opine that the number should not exceed 80. To further complicate matters, some "experts" insist that the top number doesn't matter and only the bottom one is important.

When I was a medical student, we were taught that numbers were not important as long as the patient felt well, and regardless of what the cuff read, we should not treat anyone as long as they had no complaints such as headache or nosebleed!

Well, we've come a long way since then, but a great deal of controversy still exists. For example, some doctors insist that even when the pressure is "high" by any definition, the significance of the elevation depends on where the reading was obtained—at home on your own cuff, on a machine in a supermarket, or by the doctor. Patients will tell me, "You make me nervous, doctor. My pressure is always normal when I take it in the drugstore or the supermarket. Haven't you heard of white coat hypertension?" So I take off my coat and record their pressure with my suspenders showing. The reading is usually unchanged. It's still high even when my nurse, in her *blue* uniform, records it. So they conclude that it must be the surroundings, not me. And so on.

Once everyone (patient, doctor, and supermarket blood pressure machine) has agreed that a reading is high, the next question is how best to treat it. Some specialists advocate exercise, weight loss, and reducing salt intake for as long as it takes to get results. Others say that time is of the essence and that medication should be started as soon as the diagnosis is made. When everyone concerned has decided that it's time to take medication, a whole new debate begins as to what drugs to use. It's like a medical tower of Babel.

▪ HERE'S WHAT'S NEW

Someone finally decided to clear up the confusion. In 2003, the Joint National Committee on Prevention, Detection, Evaluation, and Treatment of High Blood Pressure met in Washington and released its seventh report to the nation. Let's hope that their conclusions and recommendations will clarify all the ambiguity about this major affliction of mankind.

Here are the new criteria, in a nutshell.

Normal: Any reading *less than* 120/80.

Prehypertension: Blood pressure readings between 120–139/80–89, though strictly speaking "normal," are considered to be *prehypertensive.* These levels do not require medication, but you should start actively making lifestyle changes. This means eliminating risk factors that contribute to future cardiovascular disease, such as smoking, excess weight, poor diet (you should be eating less saturated fat and more fruits and vegetables), lack of regular exercise, and consuming too much dietary salt.

Stage 1 hypertension: Blood pressure readings of 140–159/90–99 call for treatment usually with only one drug, preferably a thiazide diuretic ("water pill"). However, if along with stage 1 hypertension you also have a weak heart, abnormal cardiac rhythm, a valve problem, or some kidney disorder in which a diuretic might be harmful, it may be better to start with a medication from another antihypertensive drug class, such as an angiotensin-converting enzyme (ACE) inhibitor, angiotensin-receptor blocker (ARB), beta-blocker, or calcium channel blocker.

Stage 2 hypertension (there is no longer a stage 3): Readings of 160/100 almost always require two or more antihypertensives, but start with one. You never know; it may be enough. Preferably, start with the "water pill," which is not only the safest but the cheapest, too.

■ THE BOTTOM LINE

I believe these recommendations are sound, and I expect that most doctors will follow them. Basically, 140/90 remains the goal for most people being treated for hypertension. However, if you're diabetic or have chronic kidney disease, your pressure should be kept below 130/80 by whatever means necessary.

After age 50, the systolic pressure is a much more important risk factor than the diastolic pressure. Keep it below 140. This is a major shift from opinions of yesteryear, when systolic pressure was ignored and diastolic pressure was emphasized.

Monitor your pressure regularly. There is no guarantee that even an ideal reading such as 115/75 will remain at that level forever. The risk of cardiovascular disease doubles with every increase of 20/10. Remember, everyone with high blood pressure has had a normal reading some time in his or her life! Even if your pressure is normal at age 55, you still have a 90 percent lifetime risk of developing hypertension in the future.

Before starting medications, try to control any risk factors you have by making whatever lifestyle changes are appropriate in your case. However, do so within a given time period, such as 2 to 3 months. If your pressure remains high despite your best efforts, start medication while continuing to modify your lifestyle. As you succeed with them, you may be able to reduce or eliminate the drugs. In the old days, only a few medications were available to treat hypertension, and most of them had adverse effects. Today, there are many more medications that are both effective and tolerable.

As far as white coat hypertension is concerned, I have a somewhat different take on it than most people. I am impressed by the reports showing that it eventually leads to the same complications as "real" hypertension. I realize that going to a doctor's office can be stressful.

I, too, get nervous when someone else takes my pressure. However, isn't life full of stress? If it goes up when your doctor puts the cuff on your arm, won't it also rise when you get your dander up at work, or experience road rage, or feel apprehensive when you hear a police siren behind you when you've been speeding? So many situations in life worry us. The doctor's office is but one. If it happens often enough, regardless of the circumstances, it can undoubtedly strain the vascular system, so it should be controlled.

Supermarket Blood Pressure Machines

IF YOU ARE BEING TREATED FOR HIGH BLOOD PRESSURE, or if your pressure is borderline and your doctor is just "watching it," measure it yourself from time to time, away from the doctor's office. Doing so is useful because some people suffer from white coat syndrome, in which they become anxious in the doctor's office and their blood pressure rises. As a result, the doctor doesn't get an accurate reading and can't know how well the condition is being treated. Also, it's useful to know your pressure in various situations, and how effectively your medication is working throughout the day.

The best way to monitor your pressure, in my opinion, is with a home blood pressure cuff. Most of these devices are inexpensive, automatic, and easy to use. To make sure the unit is accurate, take it with you to the doctor's office and check it against the one there.

Many drugstores and supermarkets now have blood pressure machines, providing a convenient, inexpensive, and easy way to measure your blood pressure. You simply slip your arm into a cuff and push a button. But are such machines accurate? Do the stores maintain their units, or do they just set them up and forget about them? Frankly, I have always been a little leery of advising my patients to check their pressure this way, especially in a supermarket.

■ HERE'S WHAT'S NEW

A nurse in Saskatchewan, Canada, who probably was also dubious of the accuracy of blood pressure measurements in these nonprofessional settings, arranged for four volunteers to test them in 16 randomly selected drugstores and supermarkets throughout the province. I was happy (and a little surprised) with what she found. Although the recorded readings were a shade high, the machines were apparently reliable using the last of three consecutive readings taken about a minute apart.

■ THE BOTTOM LINE

If you have high blood pressure, check it regularly at your doctor's office. But buy yourself a home unit so you can measure your pressure at home before and after taking medication, eating, or watching an exciting wrestling match—all away from that terrifying white coat! These home kits typically cost less than $100 and usually are reliable. Still, be sure to take yours to your doctor to have its accuracy tested against the professional model.

If you don't have a home unit, it's okay to measure your pressure at the drugstore or supermarket as long as you remember to do it three times. The last reading is the one that counts. If it seems out of line, double-check it at home or with your doctor.

How You Lower Blood Pressure Is Important

LONG-STANDING UNTREATED HIGH BLOOD PRESSURE is a silent killer. It leads to arteriosclerosis (hardening of the arteries) throughout the body, including in the heart, brain, kidney, eyes, and legs.

Fortunately, several drugs in different categories can effectively normalize an elevated blood pressure.

Is any one drug better than the others? Until recently, doctors believed that it didn't really matter which medication lowered a patient's pressure as long as the patient tolerated the drug well. Now we know that isn't entirely true. But which drug is best?

■ HERE'S WHAT'S NEW

The following shows you how important it is to keep up with medical news—almost on a daily basis. In December 2002, the results of a large study carried out in the United States were reported with much fanfare. Researchers followed the clinical course of more than 42,000 people age 55 or older who had hypertension and were being treated with different kinds of blood pressure medication. The purpose of the study was to see whether after about 5 years, besides lowering blood pressure, any one drug more effectively reduced the risk of death, heart attack, or stroke than the others.

Here's how the study was done. Researchers randomly assigned three widely used antihypertensives to the subjects: (1) Hygroton (chlorthalidone), a diuretic or "water pill"; (2) Zestril (lisinopril), an ACE inhibitor; and (3) Norvasc (amlodipine), a calcium channel blocker. To most people's surprise (including mine), although each drug lowered blood pressure to the same extent, the diuretic resulted in the lowest incidence of heart attack and stroke in patients who took it. Another plus for diuretics is the fact that they cost so much less than the other drugs.

In my opinion, the major shortcoming of this study was the failure to include a beta-blocker, such as Lopressor (metoprolol), or a combined alpha-blocker and beta-blocker, such as Coreg (carvedilol). These drugs are widely prescribed to treat hypertension as well as angina, heart failure, and rhythm disturbances of the heart. It would be important to see how they compare with the diuretics, in light of their many other cardiac benefits.

After this report, I was flooded with phone calls from hypertensive patients who had read these conclusions and who were not taking a diuretic. They were anxious for me to switch them to the "best" drug, especially considering that diuretics are much less expensive than the other drugs. I admitted that I was surprised by the findings but happy to make whatever changes were appropriate. However, I cautioned my diabetic patients that diuretics sometimes raise blood glucose levels. I also warned those who had suffered from gout in the past that water pills can elevate uric acid levels in the blood and possibly precipitate an attack of gout. I also reminded them that diuretics are called "water pills" for good reason: They make you "go," something to consider when planning daily activities.

That's where the situation remained for about 2 months, until the next unexpected research bombshell dropped. A large study out of Australia, this one using 6,000 people, found that after 4 years, use of an angiotensin-converting enzyme (ACE) inhibitor resulted in a 17 percent lower incidence of heart attack and stroke *than use of a diuretic!*

What was I to do? What was I to tell patients when there were two conflicting studies? Fortunately, an even more recent study (in May 2003) resolved my dilemma. This one did not involve a piddling 42,000 subjects like the one that recommended diuretics, or a mere 6,000 like the one that extolled ACE inhibitors. Published in the *Journal of the American Medical Association*, this one reviewed the results of 42 trials embracing 192,478 patients who were followed for an average of 3 to 4 years. The studies compared several combinations of placebo, diuretics, ACE inhibitors, beta-blockers (missing from the first study), calcium-channel blockers, and other blood pressure–lowering agents. They concluded that diuretics are the most effective first-line treatment of high blood pressure for preventing cardiovascular disease.

That settles the matter as far as I am concerned.

■ THE BOTTOM LINE

Work with your doctor to find the medication or the combination (if more than one drug is necessary) that lowers your blood pressure most effectively with the fewest adverse effects. Try a diuretic first. However, most pressures above 160/90 will require at least two drugs. The second one should probably be an ACE inhibitor. If you don't tolerate them well (they can cause a dry cough), move on to one of the others, such as an angiotension receptor blocker (ARB) or beta-blocker.

Lower Your Pressure with Sesame Oil

SESAME OIL is a vegetable oil that's good for you for many reasons. It's rich in mono- and polyunsaturated fatty acids that protect against heart disease and tend to lower cholesterol, and it is also low in dangerous saturated fats. As if that weren't enough, it contains two powerful antioxidants called sesamol and sesamin.

A few years ago, one of my patients developed cancer of the tongue. Usually, by the time this life-threatening malignancy is detected, removal of the tongue is necessary. Happily, in my patient, the tumor was still very small and localized, permitting treatment with radiation rather than surgery. However, beaming such x-rays toward the sensitive areas of the mouth and throat day after day for weeks leaves a patient painful and swollen. Swallowing, eating, and talking become very difficult.

Fortunately, this patient had attended one of Dr. Deepak Chopra's seminars in complementary medicine and heard about the use of sesame oil in such cases. She remembered learning that regularly swishing or gargling with sesame oil makes therapeutic radiation of the oral cavity much less unpleasant. She followed this advice and endured a long course of radiation without any ill effect whatsoever. (She subsequently described her experience in a written biography, and some 7 years later she is alive and well.)

I have since learned that the topical application of sesame oil to areas of the skin through which therapeutic radiation beams will pass also reduces the burning and the irritation following such therapy. I have no idea which constituents of sesame oil are responsible for this protection.

■ HERE'S WHAT'S NEW

As if all these benefits of sesame oil were not enough, researchers have found it has yet another, possibly even more important, action. It lowers blood pressure! Researchers at India's Annamalai University studied 195 men and 133 women with high blood pressure, all being treated with nifedipine (marketed in this country as Adalat and Procardia). Despite this therapy, the patients' pressures remained above normal. The patients were then asked to do all their cooking with sesame oil while continuing to take the medication. When their blood pressures were measured 60 days later, they were normal in every case.

One can't be sure what components of the sesame oil should be credited with this salutary effect. The study researchers suggest that the mono- and polyunsaturated acids lowered the blood pressure, while other experts believe it was the antioxidants that caused this benefit.

■ THE BOTTOM LINE

I'm not suggesting that you throw away your blood pressure medication, especially if it's working and you're tolerating it well. But it seems like a good idea to cook with sesame oil. It has so many other benefits, in addition to being delicious, that you may as well take advantage of its effect on blood pressure.

HIGH CHOLESTEROL

Statins for the Elderly

MIDDLE-AGE MEN AND WOMEN who take statin drugs to reduce their cholesterol levels have fewer heart attacks and lower death rates from coronary artery disease and strokes. But is it too late to take this medication in your seventies and eighties? Some of my older patients think so. "I feel fine. My high cholesterol has never bothered me, so why should I do anything about it at my age? These drugs are expensive and they can cause side effects. Why look for trouble?" Some doctors feel this way too. Are they right?

■ HERE'S WHAT'S NEW

In a recent study conducted in France, researchers analyzed the results of lipid-lowering therapy using statin drugs in more than 83,000 patients with coronary artery disease. They found that the statins reduced the risk of stroke by 26 percent when cholesterol levels were kept below 232.

In other research, 20,000 men and women who despite *normal* cholesterol levels had a prior history of heart disease, stroke, and clogged arteries elsewhere in the body, or who had diabetes, were divided into two groups. Half of them received the statin drug Zocor (simvastatin); the others were untreated. The incidence of recurrent heart attack or stroke was one-third lower in those receiving the statin drug.

In another study of almost 6,000 healthy people whose average age was 75 years and who had elevated cholesterol levels, those who took a statin drug, in this case 40 milligrams of Pravachol (pravastatin), for an average of 3.2 years had a 24 percent lower mortality from heart disease than those receiving a placebo. The total number of fatal and nonfatal heart attacks and strokes was reduced by 15 percent. The incidence of transient ischemic attacks (mini-strokes) was also 25 percent less in the treated group.

There was one surprising finding in this study. Those receiving pravastatin had a statistically higher incidence of cancer. However, the researchers point out that most of these malignancies occurred during the first year of treatment, suggesting that the subjects already had them when they entered the trial.

A study from the Netherlands is reassuring with respect to a possible link between statins and cancer. Comparing the histories of more than 3,000 cancer patients with 16,000 others, those who had taken a statin medication every day for 4 years had a 36 percent *lower* incidence of cancer than those who hadn't. However, the risk of cancer rose to "normal" within 6 months after stopping the statin. So you've got to stay with it. In this particular study, most patients were taking Zocor. I expect that the other brands would have a similar effect despite the differences among them.

There seems to be no end to the potential of these statin drugs. We know that they reduce the risk of heart attacks and strokes; they may possibly have an anticancer effect; and now there is evidence that they also protect our brains and bones. In a large study in the

United Kingdom, patients 50 years or older on statin therapy were 70 percent less likely to develop Alzheimer's disease than the untreated population. Researchers attribute this benefit to the anti-inflammatory action of the statin drugs.

Another study done in the Netherlands revealed that taking a statin drug for more than a year results in a 36 percent reduction in the incidence of spine fractures. These researchers conclude that the statins prevent bone breakdown and may increase bone density very much as the biphosphonates Fosamax (alendronate) and Actonel (risedronate) do.

■ THE BOTTOM LINE

I routinely prescribe cholesterol-lowering drugs to every otherwise healthy patient with elevated cholesterol, regardless of age, who has no specific contraindications for its use. These drugs are usually well-tolerated, but they can sometimes cause muscle, liver, or intestinal problems—side effects that clear up when the drug is discontinued.

In my opinion, anyone who's had a heart attack or stroke should be on a statin drug, regardless of cholesterol level. If you have abnormal cholesterol or a family history of heart disease or stroke, discuss with your doctor whether you are a candidate for a statin now.

HIV/AIDS

A Breakthrough Drug

AIDS IS THE MODERN-DAY PLAGUE. It affects about one million Americans and there are at least 40,000 new cases every year. Most afflicted are men between ages 25 and 44. The greatest problem is in sub-Saharan Africa, where more than one in four people are infected. Tragically, many cannot afford therapy and millions will die in the next few years.

Although there is no cure for AIDS, drugs are available that can slow its progress and improve the quality of the years a person has left. These drugs, called antiretrovirals, attack HIV and interfere with its ability to reproduce in the body. They fall into three main groups and yield the best results when used together. All three categories work by neutralizing one or more of the enzymes that the virus needs in order to multiply. When combined, they attack three or four enzymes simultaneously and paralyze the virus at least temporarily.

Unfortunately, even the most effective combination of antiretrovirals does not eradicate the virus from the bloodstream. It simply moves to another area of the body or continues to replicate at a much slower rate. Still, patients do feel better when they take these drugs and can often resume a near-normal life for a period of time—occasionally years.

The downside to these drugs is that they are potentially toxic, and as many as half the patients taking them eventually abandon them because of intolerable side effects. They are also expensive and have inconvenient dosage schedules.

One group of antiretrovirals is nucleoside reverse transcriptase inhibitors, which block the crucial viral enzyme reverse transcriptase. This particular drug is used alone only in pregnant women to prevent transmission of the virus to the infant.

The second group of antiretrovirals is protease inhibitors. They suppress the viral enzyme protease. The third group, and the most recent addition to the anti-AIDS armamentarium, is the nonnucleoside reverse transcriptase inhibitors. They inhibit the same enzyme as does the nucleoside group, only in a different way.

■ HERE'S WHAT'S NEW

In what is considered to be a major medical advance, the FDA recently approved Fuzeon (enfuvirtide), representing a totally new class of AIDS drugs called fusion inhibitors. They fight advanced HIV when all other treatments fail. This new therapy is especially welcome at a time when more patients are developing resistance to earlier treatments.

Here's what's new about Fuzeon: Whereas the older agents acted on the HIV *after* it had already infected the human cells and prevented the virus from replicating, Fuzeon prevents it from getting into the cells in the first place. Unfortunately, Fuzeon is not easy to take and is expensive. It requires two daily injections and costs more than $20,000 a year. It can also have serious side effects, such as pneumonia.

■ THE BOTTOM LINE

If you have AIDS, the right drug can prolong your life and improve its quality. There are several drugs available that are quite effective. However, when they have stopped working, speak to your doctor (and your health insurance carrier) about whether you're a candidate for Fuzeon. It may make a big difference.

Get Test Results in 3 to 20 Minutes

ALMOST ONE MILLION AMERICANS are HIV positive or live with AIDS. According to the Centers for Disease Control and Prevention, as many as one-third of them are unaware that they have it, so it's vital that you get tested if you think you may have been exposed to the virus.

Until recently, patients typically had to wait at least a week for the results of blood tests for HIV that were sent to a laboratory. The mounting anxiety as well as a natural tendency for denial resulted each year in an estimated 8,000 infected people simply not coming back for their test results.

■ HERE'S WHAT'S NEW

The FDA has approved two rapid HIV tests that require only a drop of blood from your finger. Although the first, OraQuick, was originally restricted to laboratories, it is now available for use in doctors' offices and HIV counseling centers. It is 99.6 percent accurate and provides results in about 20 minutes. The second test, the Reveal Rapid HIV-1 Antibody Test kit, gives the answer in 3 minutes. However, it's designed for use only in hospitals and clinics.

But wait! You ain't heard nothin' yet. The latest news is there is yet a third way to test for HIV—in the privacy of your own home. You get the result in about a minute! All it requires is one drop of blood obtained from a fingerstick. Simply add the blood to a blue filter and look for the color change. This "One-Minute Self Test" is sold in Monaco and 30 other countries, but not yet in the United States. The manufacturer states that it is more than 99 percent accurate and meets or exceeds the sensitivity and specificity of available FDA-approved tests. Keep an eye out for its availability in this country.

These new tests also make it possible for healthcare workers who have been accidentally exposed to infected blood to learn sooner whether they contracted the virus that causes AIDS. Pregnant women going into labor who are tested and found to be HIV-positive can now be treated in time to prevent transmitting the disease to their newborns. And if you're worried about having contracted the disease, you won't have to wait a week or longer for an answer. These tests cost about $40, and there is no public record of the results since only you and your doctor are privy to them.

■ THE BOTTOM LINE

If you think you may have been exposed to HIV, you can now ask your doctor or an HIV-counseling clinic to draw a drop of blood from your finger, test it for this infection, and give you the results then and there. No more sleepless nights waiting for an answer and fearing the worst—often unnecessarily. Even though a 1-minute, home-testing kit is available in Europe, I suggest that, for the time being, you use the two homegrown varieties sold in this country.

IRREGULAR HEARTBEAT

New Cause, New Approach

MANY OF US experience a slightly irregular cardiac rhythm from time to time, usually a harmless "extra beat"—something that does not require treatment. However, atrial fibrillation (AF) must not be ignored. It's the most common significant irregular cardiac rhythm, estimated to affect about 2.2 million people in the United States, with 160,000 new cases reported every year. (Don't confuse *atrial* fibrillation with *ventricular* fibrillation, however. The former is common and manageable; the latter, on the other hand, results in almost instantaneous loss of consciousness and ends in death if it continues for longer than 4 to 6 minutes.)

Atrial fibrillation can occur intermittently with long intervals of normal heart rhythm, but in most cases it is permanent. Although patients usually can feel the condition (perceived as an irregular pounding and sometimes accompanied by shortness of breath, chest discomfort, or both), I have many patients who were unaware that they were fibrillating and in whom it was detected during a routine physical.

Atrial fibrillation sets in when impulses that arise in the atria (small chambers sitting atop the much larger ventricles in the heart), whose job it is to direct the ventricles (the pump of the heart) to contract, go awry and fail to proceed along the normal cardiac electrical pathways. Normally, the atria generate 60 to 80 impulses per minute in a regular rhythm. In patients with AF, these impulses are disorganized, chaotic, and occur 300 to 600 times a minute. Fortunately, not all of them "get through." If the ventricles had to respond to this many stimuli, they would soon be exhausted. However, as many as 170 or even 180 impulses can reach the ventricles every minute, forcing them to contract in a rapid, haphazard way. This fast, irregular beating is what creates the symptoms that many untreated patients with this disorder experience.

Every case of AF must be thoroughly evaluated to determine what caused it—and then treated. The arrhythmia itself, when correctly managed, is not a threat to life or its quality. Most cases of AF stem from some heart "condition," such as coronary artery disease, untreated high blood pressure, one or more abnormally functioning cardiac valves (especially the mitral), heart failure, chronic lung disease, a traveling blood clot to the lungs (pulmonary embolus), disease of the heart muscle (cardiomyopathy), inflammation of the thin envelope that surrounds the heart (pericarditis), or congenital heart disease. Less frequently, an overactive thyroid gland results in AF. Other cases result from a recent alcoholic binge, too much caffeine, serious stress, use of stimulants or decongestants, severe infection, or an imbalance of body chemicals due to medications such as diuretics. The outlook for someone with AF depends not so much on the rhythm disorder as on its underlying cause.

In about 10 percent of cases, AF develops in the absence of any discernible disease, cardiac or otherwise. Some years ago, it was detected during a routine exam in a perfectly healthy astronaut training to go to the moon. It began at age 54 in one of my patients who continued to lead a normal, active life as a United States senator until he died of "natural" causes at age 86.

After establishing what caused your AF, your doctor will typically try to restore normal heart rhythm. Although there are several medications for that purpose, including some new ones, they don't always work. Your doctor may then try to convert AF to normal rhythm with an electroshock procedure, which can be done on an outpatient basis. You are given short-acting sedative or anesthetic that knocks you out for a couple of minutes. Paddles are placed on your chest, and a current is delivered to the heart through the chest wall. You feel nothing and, in many cases, you awake to a normal rhythm. It's usually successful.

If the heart rate cannot be kept within a reasonable range, you may be a candidate for an invasive ablation procedure. (The word "ablation" refers to the removal of diseased or unwanted tissue from the body by surgical or other means. In this case, it's with electrical energy, not surgery.) There are two types of ablation procedure. In one, a catheter threaded up to your heart from a vein in the groin delivers high-frequency electrical energy that destroys or inactivates the area from which the abnormal impulses originate. This leaves the heart fibrillating, but slowly. So slowly, in fact, that you may need to have a pacemaker implanted to keep it going fast enough.

The other ablation procedure delivers energy to block other impulses originating in a pulmonary vein, whose job it is to return the "used" blood back to the heart to be sent to the lungs for reoxygenation. This procedure is somewhat more difficult to do and carries with it a risk of clots forming in the treated vein. However, when it is successful (70 to 80 percent of cases), the AF is converted to normal rhythm. If you decide to go this route, make sure the procedure is done at a hospital that has a good track record with it.

If normal cardiac rhythm cannot be restored by any of the above methods, your doctor should start you on a medication to control the rate at which the ventricles beat. The goal should be between 60 and 80 beats per minute, which can be achieved by various drugs including beta-blockers, calcium channel blockers, and digitalis.

Your doctor should also start you on a blood thinner such as Coumadin (warfarin), because the greatest danger of AF is a stroke. That's because even when you control the rate at which the ventricles beat, the atria continue to beat very rapidly. As a result, they don't contract completely. Instead of blood being expelled into the ventricles on its way to the rest of the body, it just stagnates. This permits clots to form that can then enter the ventricles that squeeze them out into circulation to the brain. If you don't tolerate the warfarin well, aspirin is the next best substitute.

■ HERE'S WHAT'S NEW

Sleep apnea has been recently identified as yet another contributing factor of AF—and a treatable one at that. A study at the Mayo Clinic found that people with untreated sleep apnea are twice as likely to develop AF as are those with normal sleep patterns. When sleep apnea in patients with AF was left untreated, the arrhythmia recurred in more than 80 percent of them. When the apnea was eliminated, the AF returned in only 42 percent. Sleep apnea is treated with continuous positive air pressure that keeps the airways open during the night (see page 119).

Finally, doctors are taking a new approach to treating AF. Many now believe that it's less important to restore normal rhythm than it is to keep the heart beating at an acceptable rate and to prevent clots from forming and traveling to the brain. The fact is you can live quite normally with AF if the latter two conditions are met. So don't worry if your doctor is unable to "break" the AF.

■ THE BOTTOM LINE

If you've developed AF, consider sleep apnea as a possible cause in addition to the others described above. Normalizing your nighttime breathing may abolish your cardiac arrhythmia or make it easier to control.

Although there are many ways to restore normal rhythm in someone with AF, they are not always successful. However, remember that you can have AF and still live a virtually normal life. More important than trying to keep your heart rhythm normal is to make sure that it is not beating too fast, and that you take a blood thinner for as long as the fibrillation persists. And that may be a lifetime.

WHAT THE DOCTOR ORDERED?

NEW HOME TEST FOR CHECKING BLOOD THINNER DOSAGE

If you're diabetic, do you remember when you had to go to a clinic or your doctor's office to check your blood glucose level? Then you'd have to wait a day or two for the results—not an efficient way to evaluate the immediate impact of a meal or whatever medication you were taking to control your diabetes. Once the home glucose monitor became available, diabetes management changed dramatically. You could determine your own blood glucose levels whenever you wanted, and adjust your insulin and diet accordingly.

Millions of other Americans also need to monitor their blood regularly—those who take an anticoagulant (blood thinner), such as Coumadin (warfarin). They do so for several possible reasons:

• They have atrial fibrillation, a common irregular cardiac rhythm in which blood clots can form in the heart, travel to the brain, and result in a stroke.

• They have had a stroke (due to a hemorrhage or clogged artery in the brain) or heart attack and require "blood thinning" to prevent a recurrence.

• They have one or more blood clots in the veins of the legs that may or may not have already traveled to the lungs (pulmonary embolism).

• They have a mechanical heart valve.

• They suffer from a blood clotting disorder.

Anticoagulants prevent the formation of blood clots, prevent their spread, or both. However, thinning the blood in this way is not without risk. Unless the dose is carefully monitored at frequent and regular intervals, the blood can become too "thin" and result in bleeding or hemorrhage anywhere in the body, especially in the bowel and brain.

To prevent this complication but still take enough anticoagulant to be effective, patients must have their blood analyzed every 3 to 4 weeks. Traditionally, this has meant going to a clinic or the doctor's office and waiting for the results later that day, at which time your dosage is adjusted until the next test, 3 to 4 weeks later. This is time-consuming, expensive, and inconvenient, especially for people who travel. It isn't always easy to find a facility where the test is done accurately and results are available before your plane leaves for your next destination.

HERE'S WHAT'S NEW

LifeScan, a Johnson & Johnson company, has developed the Harmony INR Monitoring System, a do-it-yourself device that patients can use at home to determine their international normalized ratio (INR), a standard measurement of blood clotting time. It's cheaper and more convenient than having it done at some facility, and most important, you get the result immediately. Telephone that to the doctor, and receive your medication instructions there and then. The great advantage of this device is that you can check your co-agulation status as often as you want, preferably weekly instead of monthly. This should cut down on complications such as bleeding that result from blood that is too thin or not thin enough.

The Harmony monitor is available by prescription and is easy to use. You prick your finger, place a drop of blood onto a test strip, insert it (the strip, not the finger) into the monitor, and presto, in 90 seconds you have your answer!

THE BOTTOM LINE

There's no downside to the Harmony monitor. Ask your doctor about it. It's easy to use, less expensive, and oh, so much more convenient.

LUPUS

A New Treatment

THE NORMAL IMMUNE SYSTEM has "killer cells" that attack and destroy harmful bacteria, cancer cells, and other threats to the body. In a group of diseases called autoimmune disorders, the immune system malfunctions and these killer cells attack and destroy healthy tissue instead of harmful "invaders." One disorder, lupus, afflicts almost 1.5 million Americans, mostly women, according to the Lupus Foundation.

Lupus affects various organs randomly and unpredictably including the joints, heart, lungs, kidney, liver, and the vascular system. Conventional treatment, which is not always successful, consists of drugs that suppress the immune system and prevent the killer cells from continuing to go awry. The most widely used of these drugs are the cytotoxic anticancer drugs. They usually are given in small monthly doses that gradually eliminate the malfunctioning immune cells. However, this group of drugs ultimately destroys the bone marrow, so doctors traditionally removed some of the patient's marrow cells beforehand and returned them after the completed treatment to "repopulate" the marrow. This regimen sometimes works, but the results are nothing to write home about and improvement doesn't usually last long. Most patients remain chronically sick.

■ HERE'S WHAT'S NEW

Doctors at the Johns Hopkins Medical Center in Baltimore have been trying a new approach. Instead of a slow, gradual attack on the immune system, they swiftly wipe out the rogue cells with high doses of Cytoxan (cyclophosphamide), a cytotoxic chemotherapy drug. And they no longer remove bone marrow for reinjection later because some may be diseased and could make the patient sick again. Although the cyclophosphamide destroys the bone marrow, the doctors have found that the immature stem cells normally present in bone marrow are unaffected by the drug and free from disease. When treatment is stopped, these healthy cells take over and produce normal marrow.

This particular study involved only 14 patients, but researchers are optimistic about the results. About 2½ years after therapy, five patients were completely free from disease, and six had improved enough to tolerate and respond to a drug that had not worked before; only three had little or no benefit.

■ THE BOTTOM LINE

These results are so impressive that three more major medical centers have started clinical trials with this therapy. I'm reporting this news in the hope that if you, or someone you know, has lupus and are not doing well, you will contact one of these institutions and find out about participating in their study. The centers are: Drexel University School of Medicine in Philadelphia, the Medical College of Wisconsin, and Johns Hopkins Medical Center. You can also call the Lupus Center at (410) 614-1573 for more information or e-mail them at stdman@jhmi.edu.

LYME DISEASE

Don't Overtreat It

LYME DISEASE IS CAUSED BY A BACTERIUM called *Borrelia burgdorferi*. You become infected when you are bitten by a tick that has fed on an animal (typically a white-tailed deer) that happens to be harboring this bug. Most of the 16,000 new cases of Lyme disease each year in the United States occur in spring when the tick is in the nymph stage (very tiny) and less likely to be seen than in fall when it is in the larval stage and bigger.

More than half of patients with Lyme disease don't know they've been bitten and first suspect the disease when they develop the signature bull's-eye rash. This is sometimes accompanied by flulike symptoms. The rash usually persists for 2 to 4 weeks. This early stage of the disease is the best time to treat it. However, the disease may not be easy to recognize in patients who sometimes never develop the rash. If the diagnosis is missed early on, the infection can involve the joints, the heart, and the brain resulting in disabling, chronic disease.

The three most widely used antibiotics to treat Lyme disease are Vibramycin (doxycycline), Augmentin (amoxicillin), and Ceftin (cefuroxime). The prescribed drug is taken orally for 3 to 4 weeks.

■ HERE'S WHAT'S NEW

A team of researchers led by Gary Wormser, M.D., a recognized authority in this disease at New York Medical College, studied 180 Lyme disease patients. All followed one of three antibiotic dosage schedules after the appearance of the rash: (1) 20 days of doxycycline, (2) 10 days of doxycycline, or (3) 10 days of doxycycline and one intravenous dose of Rocephin (ceftriaxone), another antibiotic.

When the patients were reevaluated 3 months later, Dr. Wormser found that 85 to 90 percent of them had completely recovered regardless of the antibiotic they received. In other words, continuing the doxycycline for 20 days rather than 10, or adding the second antibiotic conferred no additional benefit. In fact, it was likely to result in a greater incidence of adverse effects such as diarrhea.

According to Dr. Wormser, "Shorter courses of treatment are safer, less expensive, and may be less likely to promote emergence of resistant bacteria that can endanger the entire community." That's because the widespread unnecessary use of antibiotics or higher-than-required doses for too long a time may result in the emergence of bacteria that are resistant to them. Several such strains of bacteria have already appeared and are causing serious, even life-threatening, infections.

■ THE BOTTOM LINE

If you live in tick country (especially rural areas of the northeast United States, Wisconsin, Minnesota, or Northern California) consider Lyme disease if you're tired, achy, have frequent headaches, and generally feel out of sorts for no apparent reason. You may have missed the rash caused by a tick bite. Regardless of whether or not you see one, let your doctor know how you feel. (The average person with Lyme disease consults as many as five doctors before the correct diagnosis is made.)

If you are diagnosed with Lyme disease in its early stages, you need a much shorter course of antibiotics than has been traditionally given. If more prolonged therapy is recommended to you, refer your doctor to the paper published in the *Annals of Internal Medicine*, Volume 138, as well as the accompanying supporting editorial by Allen Steere, M.D., who unraveled the disease in Lyme, Connecticut, nearly 30 years ago.

MENOPAUSE

Questioning Hormone Replacement Therapy

MOST RECENTLY, virtually everything that was supposed to be good about estrogen has been refuted. Mind you, there were always two schools of thought about hormone replacement. The first (and less vocal) maintained that nature must know what it's doing when it causes the ovaries to stop making hormones and thus permits menopause to set in. They advised against tampering with this normal course of events by taking hormone replacements. If nature had wanted women to continue to have estrogen, the argument went, it would have designed the female body to keep producing the hormone.

The HRT proponents scoffed at this simplistic reasoning. They argued that nature makes lots of mistakes (such as allowing cells to grow wildly and cause cancer) and that menopause is one of them. This natural error, they claimed, is why humans are one of the only mammals that develop menopause. Their solution was to replace the missing estrogen.

Over the years, there were scores of studies (most of which, in retrospect, appear to have been flawed) "proving" that HRT protects menopausal woman from a host of ailments. HRT proponents pointed out that it controls hot flashes, mood swings, dry vaginal tissue, aging skin, and brittle bones and also reduces the risk of heart disease, stroke, and Alzheimer's disease. Yes, these doctors (and I was one of them) admitted that estrogen can cause cancer of the uterus, but that can be prevented by adding progesterone. Breast cancer? We're not convinced by the data, they said, and anyway, if every woman had an annual mammogram, it would detect the cancer early enough to cure the disease. All in all, the estrogen school of thought made HRT look easy—and the evidence supporting its many benefits seemed incontrovertible. More important, millions of women who took these hormone supplements looked and felt much better.

Then came the statisticians and the epidemiologists. One by one, they proved virtually every claim about estrogen wrong. They showed that this hormone doesn't protect against heart attack and stroke but actually causes them! Doubts that estrogen contributes to breast cancer also disappeared. Its few confirmed benefits, such as reducing the severity of osteoporosis and controlling night sweats and hot flashes, were overshadowed by its many dangers.

▪ HERE'S WHAT'S NEW

One remaining myth about the benefits of estrogen—it improves memory and slows progression of Alzheimer's—was refuted in a large double-blind, randomized, placebo-controlled study in 39 clinical centers throughout the United States. The purpose of this research was to assess the effect of HRT on the incidence of dementia and cognitive impairment in women ages 65 and older. Of the 4,500 women in the trial, about half received the standard estrogen-progestin combination;

the other half was given a placebo. Researchers found that women who took the hormones for an average of slightly more than 4 years actually had twice the incidence of Alzheimer's or other forms of dementia compared with those taking a placebo! This increase translates into only 23 more cases among every 10,000 women taking the hormone. It doesn't sound like much—unless you happen to be one of them! Nor did the HRT protect against mild memory loss.

Another study of 16,000 women ages 50 to 79, followed for an average of 5.6 years, was stopped 3 years early because those receiving HRT had a 44 percent *increased* risk of stroke compared with those on placebo.

■ THE BOTTOM LINE

These studies did not involve women under 65, and in all cases, the estrogen was being taken along with progestin. Subsequent research has yielded similar results when estrogen was taken alone. All these data constitute a strong case for most women not to use these hormones. This recommendation is further strengthened by the report from the government-supported Women's Health Initiative that women taking hormones do have a higher risk of heart attack, stroke, and breast cancer.

Are there any safe alternatives to help control some of the troubling symptoms of estrogen deprivation? If you are experiencing hot flashes and night sweats, you may want to try one of the newer SSRI antidepressants, such as Paxil (paroxetine). However, do so under close doctor supervision.

Some doctors also recommend that women take natural soy products (such as tofu or soymilk) to help minimize the symptoms of menopause. Because soy contains high amounts of isoflavone, or plant estrogen, it may help protect against osteoporosis and relieve such symptoms as vaginal dryness and hot flashes. If none of the soy products help and only estrogen seems to work, take the lowest effective HRT dose for the shortest possible time. If you have vaginal problems such as dryness or irritation, use the topical estrogen creams. They appear to be safe. For the prevention and treatment of osteoporosis, there are many new drugs that work at least as well as estrogen (see below and page 195).

Evista Benefits

WOMEN WHO HAVE GONE THROUGH MENOPAUSE are at increased risk for bone loss because they no longer benefit from the protective effects of the estrogen their bodies once produced naturally. We used to think that hormone replacement therapy protects postmenopausal women against heart disease and stroke. We now know that it doesn't; in fact, it increases that risk (see page 182). What can women now take to prevent bone loss?

The drug Evista (raloxifene) is a selective estrogen receptor modulator widely used to prevent and treat osteoporosis. Although it's neither estrogen nor a hormone, it has some estrogen-like properties, the most important of which is its ability to reduce bone loss and increase bone density (thus preventing and/or minimizing osteoporosis). It does not adversely affect the breast and uterus the way estrogen does, so it does not cause cancer of those organs, tenderness of the breast, or vaginal bleeding. On the other hand it does not relieve symptoms of menopause, such as hot flashes, either.

■ HERE'S WHAT'S NEW

Data from a 4-year study of almost 8,000 postmenopausal women showed that a subset of about 1,000 women with one or more risk factors for cardiovascular disease who were taking Evista to control osteoporosis had a 40 percent lower risk of developing heart disease and a 62 percent reduction in the risk of all fatal and nonfatal strokes. (They also enjoyed a 70 percent decline in the incidence of breast cancer.)

▪ THE BOTTOM LINE

Evista does appear to exert a beneficial effect on heart disease, stroke, and breast cancer. It has few adverse effects other than a small increased risk of clot formation in the veins. For that reason, anyone with varicose veins or a history of thrombophlebitis should not use it, nor should those who are premenopausal or pregnant. However, in my opinion, virtually every postmenopausal woman at risk for osteoporosis—especially those also vulnerable to heart disease, stroke, and breast cancer—should be taking it.

MULTIPLE SCLEROSIS

Start Treatment Right Away

MULTIPLE SCLEROSIS (MS) is a chronic, progressive disease of the nervous system for which there is no cure. It is the most common nervous system disorder in young adults and affects more than two million people worldwide, women more often than men. It's five times more common in temperate zones than in the tropics. If a close relative has MS, you're at least 10 times more likely to develop it, too.

Symptoms of the disease are caused by the random denuding of the nerves, akin to the fraying of an electrical wire. The sheath that insulates the nerves and maintains their normal function becomes inflamed and is ultimately destroyed. This results in various signs and symptoms. The most common are sudden onset of visual problems, slurred speech, trouble walking, numbness here and there, vertigo, clumsiness, trembling, loss of bladder control, seizures, paralysis—in short, malfunction wherever the involved nerves are. Over the years, as more nerves become involved by the disease, patients become progressively disabled (although in about 10 percent of them, the disease does not get worse).

The cause of MS remains a mystery, but most doctors believe it's an autoimmune disease in which the body's defense mechanisms mistakenly attack and destroy healthy tissues.

Treatments for MS either act on specific symptoms or suppress the immune system and slow the progress of the disease. "Suppressive" medications include steroids, Copaxone (glatiramer acetate), Avonex (interferon beta), and others that also are used to treat other autoimmune diseases, for example, rheumatoid arthritis.

After a patient is diagnosed with MS, doctors usually wait for at least one more attack before starting treatment. (In fact, many hesitate to make the diagnosis until two attacks have occurred.) The rationale for this conservative approach is that because no cure exists anyway, one may as well delay drug treatment until the symptoms recur or are troublesome (symptoms of MS typically wax and wane).

■ HERE'S WHAT'S NEW

New research suggests that the sooner suppressive therapy is started, the more beneficial it is over the long-term. In keeping with these findings, the FDA has approved the use of Avonex, the most widely prescribed MS drug, to be given at the first evidence of the disease. Avonex belongs to the interferon beta family and is administered once a week by injection.

■ THE BOTTOM LINE

If you've had MS for some time, chances are you're already taking one of the drugs listed above. However, if you have experienced an episode symptomatic of the disease and are waiting for another attack before starting therapy, discuss with your doctor whether you should start taking Avonex *now*. It may make a difference in the long run.

New Discoveries on the Horizon

MULTIPLE SCLEROSIS is a tragic disease that inspires researchers to continue their search for even more effective ways to slow its progress, minimize its symptoms, and hopefully find a cure.

■ HERE'S WHAT'S NEW

A new class of drugs is being developed to treat MS based on the assumption that it is an autoimmune disorder. Current MS drugs act on the harmful immune cells *after* they've left the blood and begun to attack vulnerable nerve tissues. The new ones work differently. For example, Antegren (natalizumab) actually prevents the harmful cells of the immune system from leaving the bloodstream, rendering them unable to reach their target. (This unique action is expected to benefit other autoimmune disorders such as inflammatory bowel disease.) Initial observations of Antegren in MS patients have revealed as much as a 93 percent reduction in new nerve lesions and 50 percent fewer relapses.

Researchers taking another approach are evaluating the effect of the cholesterol-lowering statin drugs on patients with MS. These medications include Zocor (simvastatin), Pravachol (pravastatin), Lipitor (atorvastatin), and Lescol (fluvastatin) and their benefits seem to be endless. Although they're mainly used to normalize elevated cholesterol levels, other beneficial effects include reducing the risk of Alzheimer's, shrinking obstructive plaques in the arteries, protecting against stroke, an anti-inflammatory effect on blood vessels, and perhaps reducing the risk of osteoporosis in vulnerable women.

Now comes an interesting observation in patients with MS. In a small clinical trial involving 28 MS patients ages 18 to 55, a daily dose of Zocor for 6 months decreased the number of their relapses from 43 to 32 percent. There were also fewer new lesions detected in brain scans. Researchers presume the mechanism is the ability of this drug to inhibit several different immune responses and markers of inflammation characteristic of this disease. Statins other than Zocor showed similar effects, but they were not as marked.

It's far too early to recommend statin therapy for MS. More studies are needed—and indeed have begun—to ensure that no long-term harm exists from taking these drugs. However, the initial observations are encouraging. If you have MS, be on the lookout for the follow-up reports on this research.

As MS progresses, patients often have difficulty coping with new information and remembering it. Although usually not as severe as in Alzheimer's disease, these symptoms can be distressing. Researchers evaluated Aricept (donepezil), a drug widely used to improve cognition in individuals with Alzheimer's, to see whether it might also be of benefit in MS. This medication enhances memory modestly by increasing the concentration of neurotransmitters that help transfer messages among different parts of the brain. The results were encouraging. More than 65 percent of the MS patients tested reported improvement from Aricept, compared with about 30 percent of those taking a placebo. Objective test scores also measurably improved. Unfortunately, the drug had no effect on the disease process itself.

Fatigue is a major complaint of MS patients. A research team at the Oregon Health and Sciences University studied 69 patients with MS and reported a distinct improvement in those who participated in exercise or yoga regimens.

■ THE BOTTOM LINE

The rate of deterioration among MS patients is unpredictable. For example, I have several patients whose symptoms are barely discernible; in others, they are debilitating. However, anyone afflicted with this disease should take comfort in the fact that research is proceeding at a furious pace. New theories spawn new drugs, some more exciting than others. I have described some of the new and potential approaches that can make a difference. Don't hesitate to try those your neurologist recommends, bearing in mind that new ones will be on the way in the near future. One of them may ultimately make a difference. In the meantime, stay as physically and mentally active as you can—and keep your spirits up.

OSTEOPOROSIS

Prevent It with Vitamin D

OSTEOPOROSIS REFERS TO POROUS BONES that have become thin and fragile due to loss of calcium. The resulting fractures, especially of the hips, spine, and wrist, are a major health problem in the United States.

Twenty-eight million Americans, 80 percent of whom are women, either have significant osteoporosis or are well on the way to developing it. Among people older than 50, one of every two females and one of eight men will fracture at least one bone in her or his lifetime. Every year, this translates into 300,000 hip fractures (80,000 of them in men), 700,000 vertebral fractures (accounting for the loss of height and the so-called dowager's hump in some older women), 250,000 wrist fractures, and more than 300,000 broken bones elsewhere in the body. Pain, suffering, and death aside, all these fractures add up to an annual $14 billion in hospital and nursing home bills.

You can control some of the risk factors of osteoporosis, but not others. Here are some of the more important ones that you can't do anything about.

Sex. Women are at much greater risk than men because their bones are thinner to begin with, and they lose calcium more easily as a result of the hormonal changes that take place at menopause.

Age. The older you are, the greater your risk of osteoporosis.

Body size. Women who are small and whose bones are thinner are at greater risk.

Ethnicity. Caucasian and Asian women are at greater risk than African-American and Latina women.

Family history. If your parents had osteoporosis, there's a good chance that you will develop it, too.

However, there are risk factors you can control, such as lack of exercise, poor intake of calcium and vitamin D, especially in your early years, excessive drinking and smoking, and prolonged use of oral steroids.

Here are steps you can take that together can reduce your chances of developing osteoporosis.

Exercise. Regular weight-bearing exercise in which you work against gravity—such as walking, stair climbing, dancing, and hiking—is great for your bones and helps them retain their calcium.

Eat more calcium. One of the most effective ways to keep your bones strong as you age is to consume lots of calcium, a mineral present in a wide variety in foods. The best known dietary sources are leafy vegetables and nonfat dairy products, but there are many others. If for any reason you can't or won't eat these foods, you can get the calcium you need in supplements.

Take vitamin D. To absorb dietary calcium, your stomach must have enough vitamin D. The intake of this vitamin is decreased in the elderly, so many doctors recommend supplements containing between 400 and 800 international units (IU) a day.

If you suspect that you have osteoporosis or if you are menopausal and want to know the condition of your skeletal system, you should have special x-rays called bone densitometry. These should be done regularly every couple of years after menopause.

If these examinations reveal evidence of osteoporosis, keep in mind that several medications can halt the progress of the disease—and in some cases even reverse it. Not so long ago, women relied almost exclusively on estrogen replacement therapy to strengthen their bones. However, the downside to this hormone supplementation (especially vulnerability to cancer) far outweighs the benefits (see page 183). So you need other medications. The main ones include:

Actonel (risedronate). A 35-milligram tablet taken once a week increases the calcium content of your bones, slowing or arresting bone loss and reducing the risk of fractures.

Fosamax (alendronate). A 70-milligram tablet a week is all you need to reverse bone loss. This drug also is approved for preventing osteoporosis, at 35 milligrams per week.

Evista (raloxifene). This drug belongs to a class of synthetic estrogen-like drugs called selective estrogen receptor modulators. It shares some of estrogen's beneficial properties, such as improving osteoporosis and reducing the incidence of fractures. However, because it blocks the action of estrogen on breast cells, it does not lead to breast cancer. In fact, it may actually reduce that cancer risk. Evista's main downside is that it occasionally causes blood clots in the veins (see page 185).

Calcitonin. This non-sex hormone is prescribed for women 5 years into menopause, usually in the form of a nasal spray. It slows bone loss and reduces the risk of spinal fractures.

Any of the above is standard therapy for the treatment of osteoporosis, and all are moderately effective. However, as with any drug, some osteoporosis drugs have adverse effects, and most of the medications are costly.

As mentioned previously, your body needs sufficient amounts of vitamin D to absorb dietary calcium, so many doctors recommend daily supplements of D in doses of up to 800 IU. This is a relatively inexpensive way to prevent or treat osteoporosis.

■ HERE'S WHAT'S NEW

Doctors at the University of Cambridge in England have found that tablets containing large doses of vitamin D (the British study focused on vitamin D_3, known as cholecalciferol) taken only once every 4 months reduce the risk of osteoporosis in men and women between ages 65 and 85—and at a cost of less than $2 a year! We're talking 100,000 IU per pill, not the 800 IU of the usual daily dose. Patients so treated had an overall fracture incidence of less than 22 percent and had 33 percent fewer breaks in the most vulnerable sites, such as the hip, wrist, and spine.

■ THE BOTTOM LINE

I've never prescribed such high doses of vitamin D, but other doctors I know have—not to prevent osteoporosis but to treat multiple sclerosis, other autoimmune diseases, and some cases of advanced prostate cancer. It's unclear from this study how many of the group that received the placebo pills were also regularly taking a vitamin D supplement. If they were and the addition of these high doses in three capsules a year had such a dramatic effect, then this therapy should be seriously considered for all men and postmenopausal women with osteoporosis.

The main adverse effects of too much vitamin D are nausea, gastric irritation, and excessive calcium in the blood. High blood calcium levels can harm the kidneys and the heart. Although in this particular study, which involved more than 2,000 people, the

100,000 IU dose apparently was well-tolerated. It's still wise to discuss this new therapy with your doctor. If you decide to go for it, make sure your blood calcium level is checked every couple of months. If it rises above 11 milligrams/deciliter, forgo the next dose of vitamin D.

A Fortunate Drug Discovery

OSTEOPOROSIS is sometimes so severe that the brittle and porous bones resemble Swiss cheese. At this point, the standard treatments are not very effective, and the unfortunate patient is at constant risk for bone fracture at the slightest provocation. In such a case, a new drug may make all the difference.

■ HERE'S WHAT'S NEW

The latest medication is an injectable form of human parathyroid hormone, a naturally occurring compound that controls the absorption and loss of calcium from bone. The drug's chemical name is teriparatide; its brand name is Forteo. It dramatically reverses much of the damage of osteoporosis, increasing the thickness of bone and reconnecting the pieces by activating cells that actually make bone. In one study of postmenopausal women with severe osteoporosis, Forteo reduced spine fractures by 65 percent and other fractures by 53 percent.

Forteo is not nearly as convenient as the other anti-osteoporosis medications. Patients must inject themselves every day for a year and a half (the FDA has placed a 24-month limit on the drug's use) with penlike needles, much like those used by diabetics. The medication carries a warning that some rats injected with high doses developed a rare bone cancer. However, this finding was not observed in any of the 2,000 men and women who used the drug for up to a year and a half.

■ THE BOTTOM LINE

For severe cases of osteoporosis, where the risk of fracture with little or no provocation is great, Forteo can save the day. If you have been disabled by osteoporosis and are suffering recurrent fractures, discuss the drug with your doctor. Forteo is not for people who have had previous radiation therapy of the bones, Paget's disease of bone, or cancer metastases of the bone. Nor should it be given to growing children or young adults. However, for the rest, it may be a panacea.

Keep in mind that Forteo should be used only as last resort and only for the most severe cases.

OVERWEIGHT

The Latest News about the Atkins Diet

MANY THOUSANDS OF AMERICANS eager to lose weight are following the high-fat, low-carbohydrate Atkins Diet. This regimen has been anathema to the American Heart Association (AHA) and to most cardiologists because countless studies over the years have shown that eating large amounts of saturated fat and cholesterol for long periods of time is associated with a higher incidence of heart attacks and strokes. However, Dr. Atkins continued to insist steadfastly, until his untimely death in April 2003, that his diet neither raises cholesterol nor causes arteriosclerosis. In addition, he asserted that eating all the butter, cream, fatty meat, and bacon that your heart desires (no pun intended) actually improves the fat profile of the blood. He proposed several explanations for this beneficial effect based on the impact of his diet on insulin sensitivity and the breakdown of stored fat in the body tissues. In Atkins's view, carbohydrate is the villain, not fat.

■ HERE'S WHAT'S NEW

This past year the Atkins Diet was evaluated in several studies conducted by "establishment" scientists and reported in mainstream publications such as the *New England Journal of Medicine*. The results from one study, done at Duke University and supported by an unrestricted grant from the Atkins Foundation, are similar to all the others. The researchers randomly assigned 120 overweight volunteers either to the Atkins Diet (carbohydrate intake less than 20 grams a day, with 60 percent of calories coming from fat, supplemented by flaxseed, borage, and fish oils) or to the AHA's Step One Diet (total fat intake less than 30 percent of daily calories).

In evaluating both groups 6 months later, researchers found that subjects on the Atkins Diet lost 31 pounds, whereas those on the AHA Diet lost 20 pounds. Also, patients much preferred the Atkins Diet to the AHA Diet. Most impressive, however, was that HDL levels (the "good" cholesterol) increased by 11 percent on the supposedly dangerous Atkins diet, but remained unchanged on the AHA Diet; triglyceride levels (another risk factor for heart disease) decreased by 49 percent in the Atkins group, but dropped by only 22 percent in the AHA group. LDL levels (the "bad" cholesterol) did not change in either group, but in those eating à la Atkins, the cholesterol was altered to a form less likely to clog the arteries. Finally, those on the Atkins Diet enjoyed a 49 percent drop in VLDL levels (the cholesterol type most strongly linked to heart disease); VLDL levels fell only 17 percent in those on the AHA Diet.

About a month after Dr. Atkins died, two additional studies (one lasted 6 months, the other a year) confirmed the results of the earlier research—that is, the high-fat, low-carbohydrate Atkins Diet helps people lose weight without adversely affecting their cholesterol profile. However, at the end of 1 year, Atkins dieters regained about one-third of the weight lost, whereas low-fat dieters regained only one-fifth of their weight. In terms of actual numbers, the Atkins group lost an average of 9.7 pounds; the others, 5.5 pounds.

■ THE BOTTOM LINE

At first glance, it would appear that the Atkins Diet is preferable to the one that most cardiologists currently recommend. However, the AHA points out that virtually all the studies done thus far were of short duration. Many cardiologists remain concerned about the long-term consequences of consuming large amounts of saturated fat for so many years. So the AHA continues to warn Americans not to abandon a low-fat regimen and to follow a diet rich in fruits, vegetables, whole grains, lean meat, fish, poultry, and low-fat dairy products. In addition to concerns about vascular disease, recent evidence also suggests that a diet high in saturated fat raises the risk of breast cancer in women.

For all these reasons, until more long-term findings become available, here's what I'm telling my patients: The Atkins Diet is a safe, even healthy, short-term way to lose weight. I have no objection to overweight patients trying it for up to 6 months. However, if their cholesterol level is high or they are otherwise at risk for vascular disease, I recommend that they also take a statin or other cholesterol-lowering drug—just to be on the safe side.

WHAT THE DOCTOR ORDERED?

GASTRIC BYPASS SURGERY FOR OVERWEIGHT DIABETICS ■ Weight is a national obsession. I'd be a rich man today if I'd had the foresight to buy stock in a weight-scale manufacturing company. Do you know anyone who doesn't weigh themselves every day? My wife, my kids, and I all do. We even have two scales, one of which is set a little lower for when the fit of our clothes suggests that we've gained a pound or two, but we don't want to admit it. We aren't the only ones. Do you know anyone who isn't dieting, or who is satisfied with his or her weight, or who doesn't "need" to lose "just a few pounds?"

Ironically, this preoccupation with weight is usually not because people worry that being fat is dangerous to their health. It's mostly for the sake of appearance—you don't need me to tell you that in our culture, thin is considered beautiful; fat is not.

The truth is we're in the midst of a dangerous epidemic of obesity. Two-thirds of us weigh more than we should, and we are becoming fatter by the minute. Significant overweight leaves you vulnerable to heart disease, stroke, several cancers, osteoarthritis, sleep apnea, high blood pressure, urinary incontinence, and diabetes.

With rare exceptions, overweight is the result of consuming more calories than we burn. Mind you, some medical disorders, such as a low-functioning thyroid gland and other hormonal disturbances, can cause or contribute to it, but they're just drops in the bucket.

How do you know if you're really overweight? Most people look in the mirror or decide on the basis of how their clothes fit. Doctors used to refer to life insurance height-weight tables, but I don't know any who still do. Most men and women, patients and doctors alike, use other parameters such as the Body Mass Index (BMI) and other mathematical calculations to determine optimal weight. (Calculate your BMI using the following formula: BMI = your weight [in kilograms] divided by your height expressed in square meters.) How weight is distributed is also important: Fat thighs, for example, are safer than big bellies.

When is overweight really serious and not merely cosmetic? Doctors define morbid obesity as more than 100 pounds in excess of ideal body weight or a BMI of 40 or higher.

Everyone—your own doctor, your favorite movie star, and followers of the late Dr. Atkins—has a "foolproof" way to lose weight. Pharmaceutical manufacturers regularly churn out a succession of drugs "guaranteed" to take the pounds off—until they're forced to pull them from the market because too many people have suffered complications, even died, as a result of using them. Herbal gurus have their own armamentarium, including ephedra, which we now know is dangerous (see page 204).

Although few if any weight-reduction treatments are effective for any length of time, one "last resort" approach—gastric bypass surgery—does work. Just ask (and look at) Al Roker, the genial NBC weatherman. He's a shadow of his former self, and loving every minute of it. Like him, more and more obese people are choosing this option.

In the most common gastric bypass operation, called Roux-en-Y, the stomach is stapled and divided. It's done laparoscopically, meaning the surgeon inserts instruments through tiny abdominal incisions. The procedure seals off most of the stomach leaving a small pouch at the top that receives the food you eat. No wonder patients lose weight—the pouch can't hold very much so you are forced to eat less. Your appetite shrinks too, as does your taste for many foods. People who have this procedure require supplements because their stomachs no longer can absorb enough iron, calcium, and vitamin B_{12}. These operations result in an average loss of 50 to 60 percent of excess pounds.

Although these gastric bypass operations are normally well-tolerated, they come with the same risks as any surgery—infection, clots, pain, and (rarely) cardiac complications. Most patients remain in the hospital for 3 to 4 days after having the procedure.

One consequence of the surgery is "dumping syndrome," characterized by such symptoms as nausea, vomiting, diarrhea, abdominal cramps, flushing, and palpitations. It occurs after eating sugar because the "stomach" area in which sugar digestion normally takes place is now much smaller. As a result, sugar enters the small intestine without having been properly digested. The symptoms closely resemble those of lactose intolerance, in which lactose remains undigested in the gut because of a deficiency of the enzyme lactase. Like lactose deficiency, dumping syndrome is not dangerous, but it is unpleasant.

HERE'S WHAT'S NEW

Gastric bypass surgery offers more than just weight-loss—it can actually reverse type 2 (adult-onset) diabetes. We already know that a combination of exercise and weight loss can prevent or control this type of diabetes, but new data indicate that you can actually turn back the diabetic clock and, in effect, *cure* this disease by shedding enough pounds and keeping them off.

Doctors at the University of Pittsburgh studied 192 men and women with type 2 diabetes who had undergone the laparoscopic Roux-en-Y gastric bypass operation. Their mean weight loss was 97 pounds. Diabetes disappeared in 73 percent of them and improved in 24 percent. Only 3 percent had no change in their diabetic status. The least impressive results were seen in patients who had high insulin requirements or who'd had the disease for a very long time. But even when the diabetes was not cured, the patient required much less insulin to control blood glucose levels.

THE BOTTOM LINE

If you're overweight, and especially if you have a family history of diabetes, it's important for you to lose weight to prevent developing the disease. The best way to do that is to eat less and exercise more. But if you have type 2 diabetes, are morbidly obese, weigh 100 or more pounds than you should, or have a BMI of 40 or higher, consider gastric bypass surgery. A successful operation may improve your health substantially and even eliminate your diabetes. ▪

Ephedra—Avoid It

BECAUSE HERBS ARE "NATURAL," they are classified as "food supplements" and not regulated by the FDA. That means you can buy and consume them in unlimited quantities.

Many doctors, including myself, think that's a mistake. Why?

Many herbs are potent, which, after all, is why they're used. Some are potentially as toxic as the more than 100 potent herb-derived drugs for which you need a doctor's prescription. These are safe in small doses, but an overdose can kill you. The best example is digitalis, extracted from the foxglove plant. It's an important and powerful drug that strengthens the heart and controls an abnormal cardiac rhythm. However, if you take too much, the heart rhythm first "goes crazy" and then the heart stops. Doctors have a great deal of respect for this powerful herb; they prescribe it only in very small doses and then monitor patients closely. For these reasons the herb isn't sold in health food stores—and neither should many other herbs that are.

The herb ephedra (its Chinese name is *ma huang*) is a case in point. Until recently it was freely available without a doctor's prescription in health food stores and was widely used for weight loss and as a stimulant. It contains ephedrine, which doctors formerly prescribed as a decongestant, stimulant, and antiasthmatic but have largely abandoned because of its adverse effects. Ironically, after doctors stopped prescribing it several years ago, it found its way onto the shelves of health food stores, where it became a big seller in the weight-reduction business. Its continued use has been the subject of heated arguments between the medical profession and the manufacturers.

The first break in this war was the recommendation that warnings be placed on labels limiting the dose of the drug. That left the burden on the user. Not a good idea, according to many doctors.

▪ HERE'S WHAT'S NEW

Evidence from a recent research study in the United States suggests that people who take more than 32 milligrams of ephedra have three times the chance of suffering a brain hemorrhage (stroke) within 3 days of doing so.

In addition, researchers at the San Francisco Medical Center did a large study of all available data on the use of ephedra that was published in the *Annals of Internal Medicine*, the official journal of the American College of Physicians–American Society of Internal Medicine. They found that in the year 2001, although ephedra accounted for less than 1 percent of all herbal supplement sales in the United States, it was responsible for 62 percent of all reported herb-related complications. (Who knows how many adverse effects were not reported?)

Its most dangerous adverse effects are high blood pressure and increased heart rate, which can and do result in heart attacks and strokes. Less serious consequences are anxiety and insomnia. The researchers conclude from these data that the risk posed by taking ephedra is 200 times greater than that from all other tested herbal supplements combined! Ephedra is 100 times more dangerous than kava (which has been banned in several countries) and 720 times more dangerous than ginkgo biloba. With all the other threats to your health that are beyond your control, you need ephedra like you need a hole in the head. Researchers conclude that ephedra should either be banned or only be taken under close supervision. Practically speaking, that means making it a prescription drug available only if your doctor thinks you need it.

The ephedra saga has been evolving rapidly. State after state has banned its sale. At the time of writing, the FDA is considering removing it from the market entirely. It is possible that by the time you read this, ephedra will be no more.

■ THE BOTTOM LINE

No matter why you take ephedra, whether to lose weight or to increase your energy levels, there are better and safer ways to accomplish your goal, especially if you have heart trouble or high blood pressure. In the event that it is still available where you live, check with your doctor first to see whether you are at special risk before you consider taking it.

PARKINSON'S DISEASE

"Way Out" Treatment Prospect

MOST HEALTHY YOUNG MEN AND WOMEN have little interest in news about exotic approaches to treating conditions with which they don't identify. However, anyone with terminal cancer or a crippling disease, such as rheumatoid arthritis, Lou Gehrig's disease, multiple sclerosis, or Parkinson's disease (of which there are about 500,000 victims) is hungry for the slightest glimmer of hope for a cure. The following item should bring hope to those patients suffering from severe symptoms of Parkinson's disease—the crippling tremors, the coordination problems, the difficulty walking—all of which have been unresponsive to conventional medical therapy.

Happily, there are so many breakthroughs every day (which is what this book is about). A case in point is the following item.

■ HERE'S WHAT'S NEW

Researchers at the Institute of Neurosciences at Frenchay Hospital in Bristol, England, have just treated five patients disabled by the symptoms of advanced Parkinson's disease with growth factor delivered via a potent drug called GDNF (it stands for glial cell-line derived neurotrophic factor). It was not given orally or injected into a vein or muscle, as are most drugs. It was instead injected daily *directly into the brain through a special pump!* This technique showed promising results in rats and primates. The first objective in humans was to see whether these injections were safe. They were—and, what's more, they improved symptoms and slowed the progression of the disease in all five patients.

Even more recently at my own hospital, the Weill Cornell Medical Center in New York, my colleagues in neurosurgery have injected genes into the brain of a severely disabled Parkinson's patient. The procedure was well-tolerated, and researchers plan to perform more such injections in the months to come.

■ THE BOTTOM LINE

Injections of growth hormone, genes, or stem cells directly into the brain of a patient with Parkinson's disease are bold, new, and promising steps toward improving symptoms of this disease. Many more patients will need to be studied using these methods, for a longer period of time. However, these experiments are tangible evidence of the continued attempts to conquer Parkinson's. There is room for optimism.

PNEUMONIA

Protect the Entire Family
by Vaccinating the Kids

FOR YEARS, doctors have been recommending the pneumonia vaccine for anyone older than 65. They've also advised this vaccine for debilitated and vulnerable people of any age who might get into trouble if they were to develop pneumonia (for example, a man or woman with underlying lung disease, such as chronic bronchitis, in whom a pneumonia infection would be especially serious and difficult to treat).

Adults younger than age 65 usually are given the pneumonia vaccine every 7 years or so. If you receive your first one after age 65, no further shots are required.

The pneumonia vaccine protects against 23 types of bacteria that cause pneumonia—but many more bacteria than that are lurking in the noses and throats of healthy people. These bacteria are easily spread from person to person, and are dangerous to the very young and the elderly, and to anyone who is chronically ill.

In 2000, a pneumonia vaccine called Prevnar was approved to protect infants and toddlers against the seven most common strains of the pneumococcus bacteria. These organisms are important and common causes of various serious infections in the very young, ranging from pneumonia to meningitis. The vaccine carries a $60 cost for each of the four doses that are required before age 2. This increases the previous cost of childhood immunization by about 60 percent.

■ HERE'S WHAT'S NEW

The data are now in about the effectiveness of both the adult pneumococcal vaccine and the newer pediatric one. Here's what you should know.

Children younger than age 2 who received the pediatric vaccine (Prevnar) were 69 percent less likely to develop strep pneumonia. In children older than age 2, the incidence dropped by 44 percent. Between ages 5 and 19, the vaccine had no significant effect.

What's most fascinating is the impact that vaccinating kids has on the incidence of pneumonia in *unvaccinated adults*. Adults between ages 22 and 39—parents, obviously—had a 32 percent decrease in pneumonia when their kids received Prevnar. The incidence of pneumonia fell by 18 percent in adults age 65 and older. Grandparents, stand up and be counted! This pediatric vaccine is protecting adults by preventing pneumonia in the kids with whom they are in close contact.

The figures are not nearly as impressive for the adult pneumonia vaccine. Although it does protect against serious meningitis and was found to reduce the number of serious blood infections by half, it did not prevent pneumonia in the elderly, according to a recent study. Clearly, a new vaccine is needed for vulnerable adults, and it just may be that the pediatric vaccine is the answer. However, as this book goes to press, Prevnar has not been approved for us older folks.

■ THE BOTTOM LINE

The new pediatric pneumonia vaccine has turned out to be a blessing. Every child younger than age 2 should receive it, as recommended by health officials. It also makes it safer for us grandparents to play with our grandchildren, even if they have a sniffle that may be the forerunner of something more serious.

As far as the adult vaccine is concerned, although it isn't as effective against pneumonia, it does protect against other serious infections. If you're older than age 65, get the one-time shot. You should also get the vaccination if you're younger and you have some other disease that makes you vulnerable to pneumonia. However, stay on the lookout for a newer, better pneumonia vaccine.

PROSTATE ENLARGEMENT

A More Reasonable Treatment

"DOCTOR, I'D GIVE ANYTHING for a good night's sleep!" is one of the most common complaints I hear in my practice every day. All the clever radio and TV ads notwithstanding, you need more than a good mattress to ensure a long uninterrupted sleep—especially if you have a big prostate. Believe me, I know!

They usually have no problem in their forties, but more than half of all men have some prostate enlargement by the time they're 60, and the incidence rises in the ensuing years. By the eighth decade, 90 percent of all men have abnormally big prostates, and half of them have significant symptoms. If they're lucky, they have to get up only once or twice a night to "go"; but for many men, it's as often as every hour or two. That's something you can live with if you can get right back to sleep. If you can't, you're tired and sleepy the next day.

Insomnia isn't the only consequence of an enlarged prostate. A big gland is also prone to infection, or patients may experience urinary incontinence. When they get the signal, they have to move fast—or wear diapers.

Doctors call such enlargement benign prostatic hyperplasia (BPH) to indicate that the gland is not cancerous. Believe me, there's nothing benign about needing to dash to the john that often. (Incidentally, my brother John always referred to the men's room as the "Isadore.")

There's no way I know to prevent the prostate gland from enlarging, but you can treat the symptoms with a variety of medications. For example, drugs such as Proscar (finasteride) shrink the prostate by blocking the action of the male hormone testosterone. Herbs (red clover and saw palmetto) and a group of medications called alpha-blockers, such as Hytrin (terazosin) and Flomax (tamsulosin) can reduce frequency of urination.

Surgery for a large prostate should always be a last resort. Since enlargement of the gland occurs in various areas within it, not every case is operable. Still, more than 400,000 of these operations are done every year in this country, using a variety of techniques.

The most widely performed prostate operation by far is the transurethral resection of the prostate (TURP). The excess tissue is cut away by a telescopic "hot wire loop" inserted into the urethra of the penis. Almost 90 percent of patients improve for at least 10 years, but the operation needs to be repeated in about 10 percent of cases. The surgery leaves between 1 percent and 3 percent of patients incontinent, and at least 13 percent become impotent. There are several modifications of TURP, all of which have similar long-term outcomes.

Some patients require a more extensive operation than the TURP to relieve their symptoms if the prostate is too big, or when there are also stones in the urinary bladder. This "open" or "suprapubic" prostatectomy requires an incision in the lower part of the abdomen. It's a bigger operation than a TURP, but the long-term complications and benefits are similar.

The prostate can also be shrunk by a laser-beam or microwave procedure done through the urethra. The laser-light or microwave energy is converted to heat that steams away the excess prostate tissue. This technique also sometimes has to be repeated.

All these methods are promising and generally less invasive than a TURP—but also probably less effective. None of them is fun. That's why so many men will welcome the following news.

■ HERE'S WHAT'S NEW

Urologists have come up with what seems like a better way to get rid of a large prostate. A sophisticated laser technique, called photoselective vaporization of the prostate (PVP), became available fairly recently. The results have been very exciting. At a meeting of the American Urological Association, doctors from the Weill Cornell Medical College in New York reported that all patients they treated with this vaporization technique were discharged from the hospital within 23 hours with considerable and immediate reduction of their symptoms and no significant complications. These results, as well as those from the Mayo Clinic, have been so impressive that if you need surgical correction of BPH, you should consider PVP before trying anything else.

Side effects from this technique are fewer than those from other laser procedures because the procedure does not penetrate the prostate as deeply, so the energy it generates is not as widely spread and causes less bleeding and clotting in the tissues it attacks. In fact, I'm told the excess prostatic mass is literally vaporized, with virtually no bleeding. It appears to be the most benign and effective therapy available today.

■ THE BOTTOM LINE

Photoselective vaporization of the prostate is considered by many to be the most effective benign way currently available to reduce the size of a prostate and relieve obstruction to the outflow of urine from the bladder. It has been tested for years and sufficiently perfected to justify its use, whenever possible, for men who do not respond to medical therapy. Because of the anatomic variability of the glandular enlargement not every case of BPH is suitable for this procedure, but many are. You should consider it before submitting to any cutting operation. A word of caution: Make sure the urologist treating you has been well trained in this technique.

PSORIASIS

The Most Significant Advance in 20 Years

MALFUNCTION OF THE IMMUNE SYSTEM can cause many different diseases, and new ones are constantly being identified. The list is long and includes such different maladies as type 1 diabetes (the kind that strikes youngsters), rheumatoid arthritis, lupus, some forms of thyroid trouble—and on and on.

It's the job of the immune system to protect you against attack by viruses, bacteria, and other enemies of human health. When it spots these intruders, it's supposed to launch a barrage of defensive reactions that destroy them. However, from time to time, certain parts of the immune system apparently become confused. Instead of destroying hostile and dangerous invaders of the body, they turn against normal tissues.

Psoriasis is a case in point. It's a chronic disease that results in red, scaly, itchy patches covering different parts of the body; in some severe forms, the joints also become arthritic. Psoriasis is caused by the malfunction of memory effector T cells of the immune system, white blood cells that normally fight foreign invaders. In patients with psoriasis, these T cells mistakenly trigger other immune responses that cause the skin lesions and arthritis.

About 5.5 million people in the United States have psoriasis; in 1.5 million the skin lesions are moderate to severe. In the moderate cases, the lesions are extensive enough to involve at least 2 percent of the body surface (1 percent equals the size of the palm of your hand). In severe cases, more than 10 percent is affected.

Although psoriasis is difficult to treat and there is no cure, several different effective therapies can improve symptoms. Unfortunately, some of the best forms of therapy can be toxic or stop working after a while. The agents most widely used today are Methotrex (methotrexate), Gengraf (cyclosporine), Remicade (infliximab), and Enbrel (etanercept), as well as various ointments and PUVA (the combination of a light-sensitizing drug and ultraviolet light A). Some of these treatments also control rheumatoid arthritis, another autoimmune disorder.

■ HERE'S WHAT'S NEW

The FDA has approved the drug Amevive (alefacept) for the treatment of moderate to severe psoriasis. Amevive works by blocking and eliminating the T cells that cause psoriasis, without impairing the effectiveness of the rest of the immune system. It has been hailed as the most significant advance in the treatment of this disease in 20 years. Amevive is expected to be most useful in patients who no longer respond to conventional therapy.

Amevive is given by injection, into either a muscle or vein, once a week for 12 weeks. Patients are reevaluated after the course of therapy to see whether a second round of treatment is necessary. The makers of Amevive estimate that about 80 percent of people who've had psoriasis for more than 15 years may benefit from this treatment.

In the studies leading to the approval of Amevive, the disease did not rebound in any cases after treatment was stopped. There were few toxic reactions. The most frequent side effects reported were sore throat, dizziness, headaches, nausea, itching, and muscle ache— nonspecific symptoms common to many other medications. However, there were occasional serious complications, including blood disorders, malignancies, serious infections requiring hospitalization, and allergic reactions.

Doctors still aren't sure whether Amevive will interact with other drugs or how long patients with psoriasis should wait before using other immunosuppressant therapies after they have completed their course of treatment with this new drug.

Older people taking Amevive should be very carefully watched because it may not be as safe for them as it is for younger people. Only time will tell. The safety and efficacy of Amevive have not been evaluated in children, so it should not be given to them. Anyone with an infection or a low T cell count (for example, those with HIV/AIDS) should not take Amevive, nor should people with any malignancy or serious infection. It's not a good idea for pregnant women and nursing mothers to use it either.

■ THE BOTTOM LINE

Psoriasis can be a pretty miserable condition, not only because of its symptoms but also its cosmetic impact, especially in young men and women. Many of the drugs available to treat it are helpful. If your disease is severe and covers large and visible portions of your body and/or is accompanied by painful arthritis, try immunosuppressing agents such as methotrexate. If all forms of therapy fail and you do not fall into any of the categories I list above, consider Amevive. But make sure you're under the care of a rheumatologist or dermatologist experienced in treating this disease.

RICKETS

Breast Milk Alone Is Not Enough to Build Baby's Bones

BREASTFEEDING is obviously the most natural way to feed your infant. There are many advantages to doing so—as well as some inconveniences. If you're pregnant, especially for the first time, and haven't yet made up your mind about breastfeeding, my advice is to do it. Here are some of the pros and cons to bear in mind, and one important new piece of information.

The greatest single advantage of breastfeeding is that your milk contains antibodies against disease that your baby has not yet had a chance to develop. Breastfeeding also saves you a lot of trouble. There are no bottles or nipples to sterilize; the milk is free (whereas the cost of formula can add up over the months); it's always the right temperature; and it's right there. If you want to lose some of the weight you gained during your pregnancy, you're more likely to do so if you breastfeed because you expend about 100 to 150 calories a day just producing the milk.

The downside? Feeding a hungry baby takes precedence over everything else, no matter how you feel or how tired you are. And forget about privacy, especially if you happen to be on the subway or in some other public place. You also have to be careful about what you eat, especially if you have a family history of allergy, and you have to limit how much alcohol you drink because it gets into your milk.

Bottlefeeding has some other advantages. First of all, you can get your husband or your babysitter to take over when you're unavailable; you don't have to bare your breasts in public; and babies who are bottlefed don't get hungry as soon after "dining" as those who are breastfed because formula takes longer to digest than breast milk.

These are the main pros and cons that I can think of, not ever having had to make that decision personally. In my opinion, they add up in favor of breastfeeding simply because protecting your child against a host of illnesses outweighs all the conveniences of bottle-feeding.

■ HERE'S WHAT'S NEW

Rickets, a bone-weakening disease that results from vitamin D deficiency, is becoming more common in this country. Although breast milk contains small quantities vitamin D, it isn't enough unless the baby also spends some time in the sunlight, which stimulates the body to produce vitamin D. But these days, most parents keep their infants out of the sun because of concerns about skin cancer. As a result, some infants are at risk for vitamin D deficiency and rickets. (Dark-skinned and African-American babies are most vulnerable because their skin needs more sunlight to produce vitamin D.)

As a result of these observations, the American Academy of Pediatrics is now recommending that breastfed infants receive 200 international units (IU)—or 5 milligrams—of vitamin D every day beginning during the first 2 months of life and continuing until they begin taking at least 15 ounces daily of vitamin D–fortified milk. This supplementation should be given in an over-the-counter liquid *multivitamin* preparation. (Vitamin D supplements alone are usually too concentrated to be safe for infants.)

The Academy also recommends a vitamin D supplement for infants who aren't breastfed and who don't drink at least 15 ounces of fortified formula or milk daily. Children and adolescents who consume less than that amount, who don't get regular sunlight exposure, or who don't take a multiple vitamin with at least 200 IU of vitamin D should also receive the vitamin D supplement.

■ THE BOTTOM LINE

Unless you have a good reason not to do so, you should breastfeed your infant. However, when your baby is at least 2 months old, add a daily multivitamin supplement containing 200 IU of vitamin D. This will protect against the possibility of rickets, the bone disease that can leave a child bowlegged and too short. Such supplementation also allows you to protect your child from the harmful rays of the sun.

SEXUAL DYSFUNCTION

When Viagra Doesn't Work

IN ORDER FOR A MAN to have a satisfactory erection, his penis must receive enough blood. Viagra (sildenafil) has helped many men with erectile dysfunction, as evidenced by the 20 million prescriptions for it and the estimated one billion pills consumed. But men also must produce enough testosterone. This hormone is what gives us both libido *and* an erection. (It also helps prevent osteoporosis, depression, and fatigue.) Between four million and five million men are believed to have some deficiency of testosterone.

■ HERE'S WHAT'S NEW

Viagra works by making more nitric oxide available to the penis. This chemical relaxes the smooth muscles in the penis and widens its arteries, thus providing the extra blood needed for an erection. Researchers at New York's Columbia Presbyterian Medical Center have found that nitric oxide requires testosterone in order to function properly. When a man is deficient in this hormone, the nitric oxide released by Viagra may not do the trick. They suggest that in such cases, Viagra's potency can be restored by supplemental testosterone delivered through the skin in a gel.

■ THE BOTTOM LINE

As a man ages, his testosterone level decreases. This is a gradual, normal, and natural phenomenon that usually does not cause symptoms. A man of 80 has much less testosterone than one of 30 but can still produce enough sperm to father a child. However, testosterone levels can and often do become low enough to cause several symptoms (some call it "male menopause"), among them impotence.

If you have erectile dysfunction, get a complete medical exam, including a testosterone level test. If your your hormone level turns out to be low, ask your doctor about testosterone replacement therapy. If that does not restore potency, then add Viagra.

Viagra after Prostate Surgery

MEN WITH PROSTATE CANCER have several treatment options, depending on their age, their health, and the stage of their disease. Younger patients who are better operative risks usually choose surgery. Beyond the age of 65 or 70, some form of radiation (either external or from implanted seeds) is preferred. Older men or those in whom the disease has spread and is no longer curable by surgery or radiation are treated with various hormones. Finally, older men whose tumors are not particularly aggressive may opt for "watchful waiting" (having their condition closely followed for evidence of progression). Every one of these treatment paths, with the exception of the last, carries with it some side effects, most of which are trouble-some but manageable.

It used to be that surgical treatment of prostate cancer almost al-ways resulted in impotence and urinary incontinence. These com-plications have been somewhat reduced, but by no means eliminated, since the development of a "nerve-sparing" operation by Patrick Walsh, M.D., at Johns Hopkins University School of Medicine in Baltimore.

However, many patients who became impotent after the surgery have found that Viagra can restore satisfactory sexual performance. Incidentally, Viagra has stiff competition from two chemically re-lated drugs, Cialis (tadalafil) and Levitra (vardenafil).

■ HERE'S WHAT'S NEW

Researchers at the University of California, Los Angeles, have confirmed the effectiveness of Viagra in treating impotence resulting from prostate cancer surgery. However, they have found it to be more effective when used in a different way. Instead of taking the 50- or 100-milligram tablet 1 hour before planned sexual relations, they recommend that patients should take it regularly every night for 9 months after their operation—whether or not they're having (or trying to have) sex.

After 9 months, men so treated were seven times more likely have the same potency they enjoyed before their operation than were those unfortunate enough to have fallen into the placebo category (a risk you always take when you sign up for a double-blind study!). Twenty-seven percent of the Viagra-treated patients regained normal erectile function, compared with only 4 percent of the placebo receivers.

You might ask, why not just give these men the Viagra tablet whenever they plan to have sex? Why the nightly dosing for 9 months (during which time sex is not always on one's mind)? The researchers believe that the 9-month treatment may *prevent* impotence and eliminate the need for pill-by-pill Viagra later on. They suggest that Viagra facilitates an erection in such cases not only by increasing blood flow to the penis but also by repairing nerve damage sustained during the operation. They consider their findings to be so dramatic that they are recommending this 9-month Viagra therapy for every man who has had a prostatectomy for whatever reason and who is interested in having sex in the future.

■ THE BOTTOM LINE

Sexually active men unfortunate enough to require a radical prostatectomy should consider taking a daily Viagra tablet for 9 months after surgery to increase their chances of resuming normal sexual function in the future. Bear in mind, however, that people with heart disease who are taking nitroglycerin-type drugs or other blood pressure–lowering agents such as alpha-blockers Hytrin (terazosin) and Cardura (doxazosin) must use Viagra with caution. When combined with Viagra, these medications can cause a dangerous drop in blood pressure.

Multiple Viagra Benefits for Women

WHEN A WOMAN'S ESTROGEN LEVELS are markedly reduced, such as happens with menopause or after a total hysterectomy, she may lose interest in sex or derive little pleasure from it. For a woman motivated to do something about it, the usual treatment initially is estrogen supplementation. If that doesn't help, small doses of testosterone are often prescribed and are more effective.

Because of the impact of Viagra on male erectile dysfunction, there have been persistent rumors that this drug can also enhance sexual pleasure in women, presumably by increasing blood flow to sensitive areas in the female genitalia, including the clitoris. However, I was not aware of any convincing evidence that Viagra actually works for women, too—until now.

■ HERE'S WHAT'S NEW

Researchers at the Female Sexual Medicine Center at UCLA Medical Center in Los Angeles and Northwestern University in Chicago have made some preliminary observations about Viagra's effect on female sexual satisfaction after a double-blind study of 202 postmenopausal or posthysterectomy women who complained of diminished libido. The treated group received either a 50- or 100-milligram Viagra tablet prior to sexual activity, no more than once a day. They were screened to exclude the possibility that psychological or relationship issues might account for their problems. The participants were asked to keep notes of their reactions after every sex experience. (Now you know what your wife was busily writing the last time you were intimate.)

The Viagra-treated group reported a significantly higher incidence of orgasms than did those who received placebos. Some experienced the same mild side effects of which some men complain, namely flushing, headache, nausea, and visual symptoms.

The doctors conducting the study believe that this orgasmic response was the result of increased blood flow to the female genitals, with better arousal, sensation, and lubrication.

It is estimated that some 43 percent of women aren't very interested in sex or derive little pleasure from it—and they are not all menopausal. In many cases, it's the result of an unsatisfactory emotional relationship—and Viagra is not likely to help that. However, there is a subset of women in whom Viagra can increase the joy of sex, regardless of their hormonal status. I'm referring to those being treated for depression. One of the side effects of the most commonly used antidepressants, including Prozac (fluoxetine) and Zoloft (sertraline), is "sexual dysfunction."

Recent research results published in the *Journal of the American Medical Association* indicate that among depressed *men* on these drugs whose libido was significantly reduced, the addition of Viagra increased arousal or sexual satisfaction. The same researchers found similar results in women and presented them at the 51st annual meeting of the American College of Obstetricians and Gynecologists. They suggest that Viagra be taken at the start of the antidepressant therapy so as to prevent the decrease in libido that sometimes leads women to discontinue their therapy.

Viagra's benefit in such cases may be a placebo effect. But so what? If you're a woman who became depressed, took medication, and lost your interest in sex, there's no harm in talking to your doctor about trying Viagra.

■ THE BOTTOM LINE

If your sexual pleasure is noticeably diminished after menopause or a hysterectomy, you'll likely be advised to take some form of hormone replacement. Assuming you have no other significant symptoms due to hormone depletion, in view of all the discussion about the adverse effects of its long-term replacement therapy, you may want to consider trying Viagra first. There's no downside to it. The same is true for women of any age who have been treated with antidepressant drugs that interfered with their libidos.

If it turns out that Viagra doesn't work for you, you'll be happy to know that the money you spent on the Viagra was not wasted. Adding a small piece of a Viagra pill to the water in a vase may keep your flowers from wilting! Two scientists had previously found that nitric oxide extends the shelf life of fruits and vegetables. Viagra, like nitric oxide, inhibits the enzyme that breaks down energy-rich molecules in plants. In so doing, it keeps flowers erect and alive for up to 7 days longer. These findings were presented at an International Conference on Fresh-Cut Produce in England.

My wife has tried Viagra—on her flowers—and she tells me it works. But I haven't yet read any comments about this use from Pfizer, the maker of Viagra.

SINUSITIS

Curing Chronic Sinus Infection

IT'S NEITHER LIFE THREATENING NOR CONTAGIOUS, but chronic sinusitis is a real pain—in the head. The postnasal drip and constant throat clearing, chronic cough, recurrent headache, nasal congestion, and tenderness around the eyes and cheeks can make you miserable for months at a time.

Sinusitis is an infection and inflammation of the sinus cavities in the face and head caused by viruses or bacteria. Allergic individuals with chronically irritated and swollen mucous membranes are sitting ducks for infection. Sinusitis is difficult to cure because antibiotics have trouble getting into the closed sinus spaces. The usual scenario is round after round of antibiotics in the hope that a new and different one will solve the problem. It rarely does so—for any length of time—because of reinfection. Many patients end up needing surgery to drain the infected sinuses.

▪ HERE'S WHAT'S NEW

Researchers at Stanford University in California have successfully treated chronic sinusitis by delivering the antibiotics via a nasal mist rather than orally or by injection. They prescribed these inhaled antibiotics for 3 weeks to 42 adults whose sinusitis persisted, even after surgical drainage, and who were on the verge of being given intravenous antibiotics. The nasal mist eliminated the infection in 76 percent of cases for at least 3 months after the treatment ended. Anyone suffering from this problem will tell you that's pretty good. The results were published in the journal *Otolaryngology, Head and Neck Surgery.*

▪ THE BOTTOM LINE

If you suffer from chronic sinusitis that's hard to cure or keeps coming back, ask your doctor about receiving the antibiotic via a nasal mist. It's something you can do yourself, and it holds promise for curing the infection more effectively than oral medication.

SMALLPOX

When *Not* to Be Vaccinated

I REMEMBER how happy I was several years ago to read that smallpox was no more, that it had been eradicated forever. What a triumph for science and public health! Unfortunately, mankind was not civilized enough to take advantage of the demise of this killer agent. We (yes, that includes our own country) decided it would be wise to keep some of this lethal virus alive in a "secure location" just in case we ever needed to kill an enemy sometime, somewhere down the line. There was no public referendum on the matter—just a political-military decision. So we stockpiled smallpox virus, as did our then enemies, the Russians. Even after the end of the Cold War, both nations held onto their smallpox supplies. As they say in the New York lotto, "Hey, you never know." Our leaders must have decided that our arsenal of nuclear weapons and other horrendous instruments of mass destruction, both biological and biochemical—viruses, gases, and poisons—were not enough.

Now, years later, we have to think about protecting ourselves against this terrible disease again, not because it has reappeared in nature, but in the event some rogue state or terrorist group decides to use it to attack us. Our own smallpox arsenal is said to be secure and intact, but we cannot vouch for any deadly germs that others hold. The possibility of the theft or sale of some live smallpox virus is real enough to constitute a threat to our allies and to us.

Because the last routine smallpox vaccination was administered in this country in the early 1970s, it has been assumed that those who received it then are no longer protected. As a result, our government has made vaccination mandatory at the present time only for the military. (Our president already has had his shot.) It is recommended, but not required, for health care professionals who may be called upon to treat those infected in an attack. The vaccine is optional for the rest of the population. Whether you choose to have it depends on how real you perceive the threat to be. However, anyone who has been directly exposed to the virus must take the vaccine because the disease itself is much more dangerous than the consequences of the vaccine.

Given the renewed and widespread interest in (and fear of) smallpox, together with the fact that many people will be opting to take the vaccine, the Centers for Disease Control and Prevention (CDC) has recently updated its advice about who should not be getting it. Do not take the vaccine if you're known to be allergic to it or if any of the following apply to you:

Eczema or atopic dermatitis. Even if you had this years ago as a child, it places you at high risk for various serious, occasionally fatal skin reactions as well as encephalitis.

Other skin conditions. Any acute, chronic, or peeling skin disorder, including a burn, impetigo, chickenpox, shingles, contact dermatitis, herpes, severe acne, diaper rash, or psoriasis. Wait until the condition has completely cleared before being vaccinated.

Darier's disease. A rare genetic skin disorder.

A compromised immune system. The vaccine used against smallpox contains a live virus called vaccinia. It isn't the smallpox virus itself, but it's so closely related to it that it stimulates the same protective antibody response. Anything that suppresses your immune system leaves you vulnerable to unchecked spread of the live vaccinia virus within your body, but primarily on your skin. That includes conditions such as HIV/AIDS, any organ transplant (but not artificial joints such as knees or hips), any type of malignancy, or lupus. Chemotherapy and steroid hormones can also leave you immunosuppressed.

Moderate or severe acute illness. It isn't a good idea to be vaccinated if you're in the throes of the flu, pneumonia, or any other illness or infection. Wait until you've recovered from it.

Pregnancy and breastfeeding. Live-virus vaccination is inadvisable during pregnancy, and smallpox is no exception. Although uncommon, the risk of an adverse reaction affecting the fetus is real. Do not receive the vaccine while you're breastfeeding because it's unknown whether the virus is transmitted through breast milk.

Infants and children. Infants younger than age 12 months should not be vaccinated against smallpox, and the vaccine is not recommended to those younger than age 18 (excluding military personnel), except in an emergency.

Do not receive the vaccine if anyone in your household is also vulnerable to its complications because when you receive the vaccine, you can pass the vaccinia virus (but not smallpox) to them if they come in contact with the vaccination site or clothing or material that has been in contact with the site.

Although all doctors have been made aware of these contraindications, they are still "new" to most of us because we have not been thinking about smallpox for more than 30 years.

■ HERE'S WHAT'S NEW

The current vaccination program was formulated on the assumption that immunity from smallpox vaccine lasts only 5 years. However, researchers now believe that a person's immunity may last much longer. This new information is based on tests of people who were vaccinated as long as 75 years ago. Every one of them was found to have varying degrees of immunity to the smallpox virus. In more than 90 percent of them, the level of antibodies was considered to be high enough to prevent serious infection. That would argue against the need for mass vaccination, and support limiting vaccination to health workers, the military, and others at especially high risk.

The roughly 120 million people born since 1972, when the last shot was given in this country, obviously have no immunity to smallpox. But if you're older than age 35, and did receive the vaccine at least once, there's a 90 percent chance you probably still enjoy some protection. That's big news, and it should help you decide whether or not to be vaccinated again now.

Regarding adverse effects of the vaccine, since the current program went into effect, there have been 17 cardiac events, 3 of them fatal, associated with the vaccine in some 30,000 civilians and 300,000 military personnel. Most occurred in individuals who'd had previous evidence of heart trouble, such as angina. Although a cause and effect relationship has not been established definitively, the CDC is recommending that anyone with an existing heart problem not receive the vaccine. Doctors postulate that the vaccine results in generalized inflammation that may aggravate any underlying cardiac disorder.

■ THE BOTTOM LINE

Whether or not you take the smallpox vaccine is your decision. However, if your immune system is weakened because of any one of the conditions mentioned above, or you have a heart condition or one of the skin disorders described, do not be vaccinated. Remember that this applies if anyone in your household is susceptible to the vaccine's adverse effects because when you take the vaccine, you become a "carrier" as far as they are concerned.

In my own practice, I am recommending it only for those patients who are health care workers or likely for some other reason to be in close contact with an infected person in the event of a terrorist attack. I do not plan to take it myself because I am counting on the immunity I enjoy from my last shot some 35 years ago.

Having said all that, let me emphasize two key points. First, if you choose not to have the vaccine at this time for any reason and terrorists attack with the virus, there is a window of about 4 days after exposure during which you can be vaccinated and protected. Second, even if you have any condition that precludes being vaccinated now in the event of a *future* attack, you will have to be vaccinated if and when such an attack occurs.

Donating Blood after Vaccination

THE GOVERNMENT HAS RECOMMENDED that some Americans be vaccinated against smallpox because of a possible terror attack. Many individuals at greatest risk (health care providers and military personnel) have already received the vaccine that contains the live virus. For the moment, smallpox vaccination remains optional for the rest of the population and is not recommended at this time because its risks may outweigh its benefits.

▪ HERE'S WHAT'S NEW

If you recently have been vaccinated and are thinking of donating blood, you must take certain precautions. Why? Because the vaccine you were given contains a live virus that can be transmitted to anyone who receives your blood. So don't donate (other than to yourself) for at least 3 weeks after getting the shot or until the scab at the injection site falls off, whichever is later. If you experienced an adverse reaction to the vaccine, delay giving blood for at least 14 days after that reaction has cleared up. If you aren't asked about smallpox vaccination at the blood bank, be sure to volunteer this information.

■ THE BOTTOM LINE

Hold off on donating your blood for at least 3 weeks after being vaccinated for smallpox, because the live vaccine it contains can be transmitted to a blood recipient, who may not be able to tolerate it.

STROKE

Prevention: Something Old, Something New

DESPITE ALL THE NEW SOPHISTICATED TECHNOLOGY to diagnose whatever ails you, the old-fashioned stethoscope remains an important tool. Unfortunately, doctors use it less and less these days. They either leave it in a coat pocket with just enough showing as their "ID" or, what's even more chic, they drape it around the neck. Who needs a necktie with such professional attire?

Besides using the stethoscope to examine your heart and lungs, it's important for your doctor to place it over the arteries in your neck to listen for a *bruit* (pronounced *broo-ee*). A bruit is the sound generated by blood flowing through a narrowed artery, in this case the carotids that carry the blood from the heart through the neck into the brain. When one or both of these arteries are significantly narrowed, you are at risk for having a stroke. What a simple, inexpensive way to detect a life-threatening condition!

If your doctor hears a bruit, the next step is to order a carotid sonogram. That's also simple to do, but a lot more expensive. It determines the degree of blockage so that you and your doctor can decide whether anything needs to be done about it. The loudness of the bruit does not always reflect the severity of the obstruction. In other words, a soft sound may reflect a serious problem whereas a loud one may not. However, *every bruit requires evaluation*.

If the obstruction is found to be "high grade"—that is, severe enough to warrant removal—there are two ways to do so. The first is called a carotid endarterectomy, in which the obstructing plaques in the arterial wall are surgically scraped away. A newer, nonsurgical technique balloons open the artery and then keeps it open with a sleeve called a stent. This is similar to the technique used to open diseased coronary arteries in the heart.

■ HERE'S WHAT'S NEW

Over the years, doctors have been compiling statistics to compare the safety and efficacy of surgery and stenting of carotid artery blockages as opposed to "watchful waiting." The results are now in. Stenting wins hands down as the procedure of choice for patients at high risk. What has made the difference is the use of an ingenious little "umbrella" (called an Angioguard) that's inserted into the neck artery before the stenting procedure. It traps any debris or little pieces of the plaques that may break off during the procedure, so they don't travel up to the brain and cause a stroke. After the stenting is finished, the umbrella is removed.

This combination of stent and the Angioguard has reduced many of the complications of surgery in carotid artery obstruction in high-risk patients. Here's how results with both techniques compare: Thirty days after each procedure, the rate of stroke, heart attack, or death in the stented group was 5.8 percent; in those treated surgically, it was 12.6 percent. As far as strokes are concerned, the incidence in stented patients was 3.8 percent; in the surgical group, 5.3

percent. The risk of heart attacks was 2.6 percent versus 7.3 percent. Stenting is safer in every respect.

▪ THE BOTTOM LINE

Always make sure your doctor listens carefully to your neck during a routine physical examination. Carotid blockages usually don't cause symptoms—your doctor must listen for them. If he or she hears an abnormal sound (a bruit), you should be further tested with a carotid sonogram. If that reveals a blockage severe enough to require correcting, ask your doctor how it will be done. If the answer is surgical endarterectomy, ask about the stenting procedure. It may not be offered as an option because it's relatively new and not done in every hospital. This also is a good time to ask for a second opinion from a specialist with experience in carotid stenting.

Can You Recognize the Signs of a Stroke?

IT'S INCREDIBLE BUT TRUE: Most people with symptoms of a stroke severe enough to send them to hospital don't know the cause of their illness until they've been told the diagnosis. They honestly don't understand what their symptoms mean. This is also true of bystanders and family members. Stroke education is important because interpreting the symptoms quickly and getting to the hospital as soon as possible permits early treatment that can reduce the long-term complications of what doctors call a "cerebrovascular accident."

▪ HERE'S WHAT'S NEW

Researchers at the University of North Carolina in Chapel Hill created a script to be used by bystanders, family members, and patients to alert them to the possibility of a stroke. Of course, if you haven't a clue that someone is having a stroke, the following won't help. However, if you suspect a stroke, ask the person to do three simple things:

1. Smile

2. Raise both arms and keep them up

3. Speak a simple sentence

The inability to carry out any one of these commands is the most common indication of a stroke. Attempts to smile result in obvious facial distortion because the facial muscles are weakened or paralyzed. A stroke patient may not be able to raise an arm because it also has been weakened. And the patient may have slurred or unintelligible speech.

You might be wondering where the researchers found enough subjects to evaluate this simple test. You can't stand in the street waiting for lots of people to have strokes. And you don't want to wish one on yourself. The researchers came up with an ingenious answer: Why not find some volunteers to test it on hospital patients who had recently had strokes? That's what they did. (I must say that these researchers had a little chutzpah. If I were in a hospital recovering from a stroke, I wouldn't welcome a bunch of strangers coming to my bedside and asking me to smile!)

The test itself had two goals: First, to see whether the average layman would be able to administer and interpret the results. Second, to determine whether the symptoms tested really appear often enough in a stroke.

Here's what the researchers found: Of the 100 selected volunteers, 96 were able to administer the test properly. They detected arm weakness 95 percent of the time, facial weakness 71 percent of the time (I suppose that's because even normal faces can be asymmetrical), and slurred speech in 88 percent of patients. That's pretty good. I mean, we aren't exactly doing MRIs and CT scans of the brain!

■ THE BOTTOM LINE

Learn and apply these three simple steps when you or anyone else suddenly develops symptoms that raise the possibility of a stroke. If one or more are abnormal, get yourself or them to the hospital ASAP.

THYROID CANCER

Radiation Exposure and Potassium Iodide

SINCE SEPTEMBER 11, 2001, Americans have been conditioned to expect other terrorist attacks. One of the fears is about radiation exposure either from a nuclear attack or contamination from a faulty nearby nuclear facility.

Unfortunately, nothing will protect you if you're near ground zero and you receive a megadose of radiation. But if you do survive, you're at risk for thyroid cancer years later. That's what happened in Chernobyl when its power plant suffered a major leak. Most of the victims were kids who later developed thyroid cancer.

■ HERE'S WHAT'S NEW

The American Academy of Pediatrics is recommending that households, schools, and child care centers within 10 miles of a nuclear power plant keep potassium iodide pills on hand to protect children from accidental or intentional release of radiation. The

Academy suggests stockpiling these pills even within a larger radius because of fallout that could be carried a greater distance downwind, such as that which occurred near Chernobyl.

Federal nuclear regulators have made potassium iodide available free of charge to states with nuclear plants, and these states have provided them to citizens deemed geographically vulnerable. Also, the U.S. Nuclear Regulatory Commission requires nuclear plants to stockpile potassium iodide to protect plant workers.

Potassium iodide blocks the thyroid gland's absorption of harmful radioactive iodine, which can cause cancer in the future. Children are more vulnerable to thyroid cancer from radioactive iodine in fallout because their glands absorb and metabolize iodine more easily. When the children take potassium iodide pills, the iodine they contain is picked up by the thyroid, rendering the gland unable to handle any more when iodine presents itself in radioactive form.

■ THE BOTTOM LINE

If you live within 15 miles of a nuclear plant, no one will think you're neurotic if you stock up on some potassium iodide, especially if you have children in your household. It's best to play it safe, especially when it's so easy—and free. I'll let you in on a little secret: We have no kids at home anymore, but guess what? I keep a bottle of potassium iodide in our medicine chest.

These pills do not require a prescription, they have few if any adverse effects, and you can get them at a drugstore or on the Internet. If you don't open the bottle and keep it at room temperature, the pills maintain their potency indefinitely. They work best when taken immediately after exposure. The dose is 130 milligrams for anyone who weighs more than 154 pounds; those who weigh less should take half that amount. The recommended dose for children up to

1 month of age is 16 milligrams; for children 1 month to 3 years of age, it's 32 milligrams.

Taking thyroid supplements does not interfere with this pill. One dose of potassium iodide provides 24 hours of protection, by which time you should have hightailed it out of the area. Radioactive iodine remains in the environment for 8 days, so once you leave, you should stay away from home for at least that long. If you can't or won't leave, take the pills until significant risk of exposure to radioiodines no longer exists.

URINARY TRACT INFECTION

More Juice, Less Sex!

ABOUT 10 MILLION AMERICANS, most of them women, develop a urinary tract infection (UTI) every year. In many, the problem is recurrent. Men also suffer from UTIs, but much less frequently. There are several reasons for this difference. First, the urethra, the duct that carries the urine out of the body, is much shorter in women and its opening is close to the anus and vagina, both of which harbor the most common UTI-causing bacteria, *Escherichia coli*. Women who use a diaphragm are more vulnerable to UTI as a result of sexual intercourse. The risk of infection is even greater if their partner uses a condom with a spermicidal foam. These foams promote the growth of *E. coli*.

Menopausal women who lack estrogen develop thinner tissue in the vagina, urethra, and bladder that makes them vulnerable to irritation and infection. Diabetics are also more prone to UTIs because bacteria thrive in the glucose of the urine. So are children younger than age 2, whose soiled diapers are loaded with bacteria. Men who require catheterization because of prostate enlargement or for other reasons are also susceptible to UTIs.

Treating recurrent UTIs first and foremost consists of removing the offending cause. Then several antibiotics can eradicate these infections. Drinking lots of fluids and avoiding alcohol also helps.

■ HERE'S WHAT'S NEW

Frankly, much of the following is not really new but does reinforce with impressive data what most people already suspected. For example, it's no secret that cranberry juice helps prevent recurrent UTIs. The news is that juice from many other kinds of berries also works. So if cranberry juice is not your cup of tea, you can also drink fresh juice from blueberries, raspberries, strawberries, lingonberries (I don't know anyone who's ever had lingonberry juice), cloudberries (ditto), and currants. Other fruit juices (apple, orange, grapefruit) are useful too, but not to nearly the same extent as berry juices. Researchers at the University of Finland, found that whereas one glass of fruit juice (up to a maximum of three a day) reduced the incidence of UTIs in women by one-third, berry juices did so twice as often.

Berries work because they are rich in flavonols, compounds that make it hard for the germs in the urinary tract to hold on to the body's cells. As a result, they are washed away with the urine (the bacteria, that is, not the cells!).

It isn't only what you drink that's important. Certain foods such as sour cream, live-culture yogurt, and cheese are also helpful because they contain friendly bacteria that replace the harmful ones. Women who consume them at least three times a week have only one-fifth the incidence of UTIs than those who don't.

All of which brings us to the matter of sex. I wish I had better news for you. The more sex a woman has, the more vulnerable she is to UTIs. Specifically, having sexual intercourse a minimum of three times a week triples the risk as compared to once a week. This is the kind of prescription doctors don't like to give. Do with it what you will.

■ THE BOTTOM LINE

If you're prone to urinary tract infections, whether you're male or female, first eliminate any obvious cause. Diabetics should keep their blood glucose level under optimal control. Menopausal women may need vaginal estrogen suppositories to reduce dryness and irritation (they do not carry the risk of the oral preparations). Women should consider personal hygiene (something as obvious as wiping *away* from the vagina after a bowel movement). And learn to recognize the symptoms of a UTI so you can nip the infection in the bud with the appropriate antibiotics.

Then there's the matter of diet. Get into the habit of drinking some kind of berry juice at least three times a week, eating yogurt two or three times a week, or both.

As far as sex is concerned, continue to use condoms by all means, but avoid those that are coated with potentially irritating spermicides. And change from a diaphragm to another form of birth control. How often you have sex is entirely up to you. Personally, I wouldn't cut down. It isn't worth it!

UTERINE FIBROIDS

Avoid or Delay Surgery

UTERINE FIBROIDS are the most common benign tumors in women. They occur at any age in 25 percent of all females, usually before menopause, and are the leading reason for having a hysterectomy. Whether they cause symptoms (they do in about 40 percent of women older than age 35) depends on their number and how big they become. They can be as small as a pea or larger than a cantaloupe; they may be single or numerous.

Fibroids require treatment only if their symptoms warrant it. If there are too many or they are too big, they may cause heavy menstrual bleeding, pelvic or lower back pain, frequent urination, a swollen or distended abdomen, pain or trouble moving your bowels, and difficulty becoming or staying pregnant.

Current treatment of fibroids includes:

Hormone therapy. Fibroid development may be related to a woman's estrogen levels, and reducing these levels in the body can decrease the size of the tumors.

Myomectomy. This surgical procedure removes only the fi-broids, 10 to 30 percent of which recur. It is possible for a woman to become pregnant after a myomectomy, but the procedure may affect fertility if the uterus is scarred.

Hysterectomy. This is major surgery in which the uterus is re-moved, resulting in infertility.

Fibroid embolization. This invasive but nonsurgical procedure is done using a local anesthetic and allows the patient to go home the same day. A tiny catheter is introduced into an artery reached through a small incision in the thigh. Microparticles injected through the catheter into the artery end up in the blood vessels that supply the fibroid, blocking these "feeder" vessels, starving and thereby shrinking the fibroid. Embolization has a 94 percent success rate in experienced hands; some patients remain fertile if they are premenopausal and the uterus is not cut, scarred, or removed.

■ HERE'S WHAT'S NEW

There are some new observations about the embolization tech-nique. Doctors at the University of Toronto found that among 555 women with fibroids who had this procedure and who hoped to have babies someday, 14 went on to do so within 2 years. Although that figure isn't high, remember that the hysterectomy alternative would have meant no babies at all.

There is news on the drug front as well. Mifepristone, better known as RU-486 (the so-called abortion pill), was approved by the FDA in 2000 for inducing abortion during the first 7 weeks of preg-nancy. This drug has now been shown to shrink fibroids, too.

Doctors at the University of Rochester in New York found that as low a daily dose as 5 milligrams (600 milligrams are usually needed to cause abortion) can halve the size of fibroids within 6 months. At the same time this treatment improves such symptoms as bladder pressure, and pelvic and low back pain. Although higher doses of

RU-486 can cause hot flashes, these are not as common with 5 milligrams a day.

■ THE BOTTOM LINE

Treatment with RU-486 may be a good idea for women whose fibroids are enlarging but who do not require urgent intervention—for example, if they are not bleeding heavily and becoming progressively more iron deficient. Try to hold out until menopause when fibroid growth slows down, reducing the need for hysterectomy. However, if more invasive therapy is required and you can't wait, I suggest you look into the embolization technique. If you're of childbearing age and want to have babies, your best choices to deal with the fibroids are myomectomy and embolization.

WRINKLES

A New Wrinkle with Botox

BOTOX IS THE COSMETIC RAGE THESE DAYS, especially to remove the wrinkles that let people know how you really feel (I prefer to call them "scowl lines"). These injections work. I have seen their results on the faces of so many beautiful people who apparently never get angry.

■ HERE'S WHAT'S NEW

Dermatologists at the Weill Cornell Medical College have noticed that new wrinkles have appeared in some patients whose original wrinkles were successfully eliminated with Botox. Here's how and why it happens. According to the Cornell doctors, when a patient unwittingly scowls, nearby muscles in the upper nose, middle eyebrow, and eyelid are called into play because the original ones were paralyzed in order to remove the wrinkles. The involvement of these alternative muscles, if it occurs often enough, may create new wrinkles.

■ THE BOTTOM LINE

Botox injections must be repeated every few months. So in the weeks and months after your first treatment, examine your face carefully. If you see new wrinkles in previously unaffected areas, you have two choices: Don't bother getting more shots (they don't come cheap), or be prepared to have the newly involved new areas "Botoxed," too.

EPILOGUE

At this point, Bugs Bunny would have said, "That's all, folks." But he'd have been wrong, for there's no end to medical discoveries that make the difference between life and death or that enhance our existence.

However, in the real world, we must consider publishing deadlines. Were it not for them, I could have gone on writing, day after day, about all the wonderful and interesting findings that constitute *Breakthrough Health*.

Given these practical constraints, I have continued searching for breaking medical news up to the last moment before this book went to press. I have reported the latest information as a series of bulletins in the section called "Hold the Presses!" that begins on page 263. And I have decided that this book will the first of many volumes in my goal to report to you the saga of practical medical research, ongoing observations, and discoveries that you can use.

Along with lots of brand-new information, look for in-depth analysis of this year's bulletins in *Breakthrough Health 2005*. I'll let you know what has stood the test of time and what hasn't, and I'll provide relevant updates based on the newest research.

My goal is to keep you, my readers (all of whom I view as if you were my own patients), up to date on what's new and worthwhile in the field of human medicine. I expect to do so for as long as I can and for as long as you keep reading what I've written.

May every one of you find something in the foregoing pages that has made a difference to your health and well-being. Stay with it. It should be fun—and important.

HOLD THE PRESSES!

More red wine benefits. New research from Harvard suggests that red wine in moderation prolongs life by about 70 percent—at least in worms and fruit flies. This beneficial effect is presumed to be caused by resveratrol, a compound in the skin of the grape (and, incidentally, also in peanuts) that acts on other proteins to slow down or prevent cell death. The next step is to test these observations in rodents and eventually in humans.

Fish safety. Researchers at Stanford University, using newly available x-ray technology, have observed that the mercury in the muscle of fish is different and possibly less harmful than any of the other 26 known mercury compounds, each with its own toxicity profile. Scientists are cautiously optimistic that mercury in fish will be cleared of its present stigma, but they caution not to act yet on these initial observations.

Herpes help. The antiviral drug Valtrex (valacyclovir) substantially reduces the severity and duration of herpes infection as well as the incidence of its recurrence. The FDA has approved claims by the drug's manufacturer that it also decreases the chance of spreading the herpes infection to one's sexual partner by about 50 percent. Patients are still advised to avoid sexual contact during the characteristic flare-ups when sores reappear and to use condoms, although neither approach is foolproof.

Calcium to avenge Montezuma. Researchers in the Netherlands have found that subjects who were infected with a strain of *Escherichia coli*, the most common culprit in traveler's diarrhea, and received dietary calcium supplementation recovered 1 day sooner from their infection than did a control group. Their diarrhea was also less severe, and they lost less weight.

Mind over nausea. Researchers at the University of Rochester Medical Center evaluated acupressure wristbands for their effectiveness in controlling nausea in 700 cancer patients receiving chemotherapy. The wristbands had no effect on the nausea unless the patients expected them to be of help.

Botox for big prostates. Italian researchers injected Botox directly into the prostate glands of 15 men with symptoms of prostate enlargement. Men in a similar group were given placebo injections of saline. After 2 months, symptoms were reduced by 65 percent in 13 of the 15 Botox recipients. Only three of those who received the placebo said they felt better.

Another ACE inhibitor benefit. British researchers believe that people with uncomplicated coronary artery disease should take an angiotensin-converting enzyme (ACE) inhibitor in addition to a daily aspirin and a statin drug. They found that 12,000 patients given one of these medications had a 20 percent lower risk of cardiovascular death, heart attack, and cardiac arrest during the 4 years they were monitored. These doctors believed that adding the ACE inhibitor would prevent 100,000 heart attacks in their country with its population of 60 million.

Is your headache really migraine? Researchers at the Albert Einstein College of Medicine in New York have come up with three simple questions to help you identify whether your headache is a migraine. If you answer "yes" to two of the three questions, chances are you have a migraine. The questions are: 1) Has a headache limited your activities for a day or more in the last 3 months? 2) Are you nauseated or sick to your stomach when you have a headache? 3) Does light bother you when you have a headache?

A UTI vaccine. Researchers at the University of Wisconsin Medical School have developed what they call "vaginal mucosal immunization" to prevent recurrent urinary tract infections in women. This vaccine takes the form of a vaginal suppository and may help prevent the emergence of antibiotic-resistant bacteria.

New uterine fibroid treatment. Doctors at five hospitals around the world including the Brigham and Women's Hospital in Boston have aimed ultrasound beams from outside the body to destroy fibroids. Patients require little pain medication, and they can go home the same day and return to work within a couple of days. This ultrasound technique looks promising, but it is still experimental. Doctors are not sure whether the fibroids will come back.

Good news for senior insomniacs. Researchers in the United States are enthusiastic about a new sleep medication called eszopiclone. (I am sure that its trade name, when announced, will be easier to remember and pronounce.) They found a 2-milligram dose to be effective, particularly in older people with a chronic sleep problem. It improved the quality and depth of slumber and increased the total sleep time. What's more, those who did awaken for any reason went back to sleep much more quickly.

A 3-minute hysterectomy. The FDA recently approved an amazing new alternative to hysterectomy. It's called microwave endometrial ablation and can be done as an outpatient procedure under light anesthesia. It involves using a handheld wand to emit high-frequency microwaves. It's fast (it takes 3 to 5 minutes), safe, and an effective alternative to surgery.

When to take Proscar. Recent research involving 19,000 men ages 55 and older at the University of Texas Health Sciences Center has shown that Proscar (finasteride), a drug used to treat symptoms of prostate enlargement, reduces the incidence of prostate cancer by nearly 25 percent. However, the drug did have a downside. Researchers observed that the cancers prevented by Proscar were small, probably insignificant ones, but that the number of life-threatening aggressive cancers increased.

Men, loosen your ties! British researchers reported in the *British Journal of Ophthalmology* that wearing a necktie too tight may increase the chance of developing glaucoma, an important cause of vision loss. In their experiments, these doctors found that tightening the tie raised eye pressure in 60 percent of men with glaucoma and 70 percent of normal males.

Medicare will pay for emphysema surgery. For people with advanced cases of emphysema, surgical removal of a portion of the diseased lung greatly improves quality of life. The average cost of such surgery and follow-up is $61,000. Medicare has announced that the benefit of such surgery is enough for them to pick up the tab, which is good news for those unable to afford the procedure on their own.

When to change hospitals. Suppose you suddenly develop chest pain due to a heart attack and you immediately go to the nearest emergency department. The treatment you receive will depend on what that particular hospital can deliver. There are two main choices. You can be given clot-busting drugs or have a balloon angioplasty, in which the fresh clot is removed opening the blocked artery. Recent research reported in the *New England Journal of Medicine* indicates that 14 percent of heart attack patients treated with clot-busting drugs either died, or had another heart attack or stroke within 30 days, compared with only 8 percent treated with angioplasty.

Unfortunately, only 15 percent of hospitals in this country have the catheterization laboratory needed to perform this procedure. The location of such a hospital nearest you is the kind of information you should have before an attack occurs. If you have the choice, that's where you should ask the ambulance crew to take you. One important finding in this study was that patients who were transferred for angioplasty *within 2 hours* had the same benefit as those who had it immediately.

Statins for your eyes, too. The combination of aspirin and a statin is an effective way to reduce your chances of developing a form of macular degeneration. Researchers at the University of California School of Medicine in San Francisco found that people who had taken a statin drug were 60 percent less likely to develop this eye problem (and were also 60 percent more likely to have been on a daily aspirin).

New treatment for interstitial cystitis? This chronic condition causes severe bladder pain in many women. A small study suggests that injecting a solution containing a bacterium called BCG into the bladder reduces symptoms in nearly 70 percent of patients.

Ban chromium picolinate? The Food Standards Agency, a group of independent scientists and doctors that advises the British government, has called for a ban on the supplement chromium picolinate on the grounds that it can cause cancer of the upper respiratory tract, lungs, and stomach. Chromium picolinate is widely used by athletes, body builders, and diabetics. However, according to a more recent study of people with type 2 diabetes, adding 1,000 micrograms of chromium picolinate to their diet increased their insulin sensitivity by almost 9 percent. No mention of the cancer issue was made in this new research.

Chelation for stented arteries. Coated stents placed in arteries that have been ballooned open reduces the incidence of their closure—but they're expensive. Copper chelation may provide a cheaper and even more effective solution.

No spuds during pregnancy? Researchers in Australia have found that harmful bacteria present in soil can infect potatoes and beets. When pregnant women who are genetically vulnerable to diabetes eat these foods, the bacteria they contain can destroy the insulin-producing cells of their newborn and cause diabetes.

Other effects of NSAIDs. It's well known that anti-inflammatory drugs such as Advil (ibuprofen) can cause stomach irritation and bleeding. Now, thanks to a new disposable little camera that you can swallow and that takes pictures as it travels down the intestinal tract, nonsteroidal anti-inflammatory drugs (NSAIDs) have been shown to affect the small intestine in the same way.

Calming "restless legs." Restless leg syndrome is a neurologic disorder that affects up to 10 percent of the population. It interferes with sleep and causes pain as well as an uncontrollable urge to move the legs. A new drug called Requip (ropinirole) significantly improves symptoms and is well-tolerated.

Carotid artery decision. Some plaques in the carotid arteries (in your neck) should be removed to prevent a stroke; others can safely be left alone. It's been the doctor's judgment call—until now. Early study results suggest that an MRI of the neck may be able to distinguish between those that can cause trouble and those that won't.

Nuts to you! Previous studies have shown that eating almonds improves your cholesterol and related blood levels. But the surprise is that despite their high energy content, almonds are not likely to cause weight gain. That's presumably because they promote increased excretion of fat in the stool.

Microwave those dentures. Just brushing and cleaning your dentures does not rid them of the bacteria and fungi that can cause sores and infections of the gums and mouth. You need to microwave them. If they have no metal components, put them in a microwave container with vents, add a denture cleaner, cover them with a towel, microwave them for 2 minutes, then cool and rinse.

The latest migraine medication. The "triptans" are the latest, most effective medications for migraine. There are differences among them in terms of adverse effects and duration of action. Frova (frovatriptan), the latest one approved by the FDA, is said to have fewer adverse effects and remains in the blood for about 26 hours longer than any other triptan.

Warts away! Your kids will be happy with this one. The common warts so many of them have can now be removed by an over-the-counter aerosol spray that freezes them. Most warts then fall off within 10 days. If they don't, simply spray them again. No more visits to the dermatologist for liquid nitrogen.

Good bacteria for ulcerative colitis. If you're one of the 500,000 Americans with chronic ulcerative colitis, an inflammatory bowel disease (the other is Crohn's disease), a novel treatment has been shown to be effective. VSL#3 is a combination of 450 billion harmless bacteria (such as lactobacillus), which, taken by mouth, helps balance the intestinal bacterial population that may be infecting and inflaming your gut. In a recent trial, 86 percent of 30 patients with this problem responded to this treatment.

Keep your nitroglycerin. Doctors have always told their patients that nitroglycerin tablets (the little white pills that are used to treat angina and dissolve under the tongue) should be discarded 6 months after the bottle has been opened. That's no longer necessary. The pills have now been reformulated so you can keep them until the expiration date on the bottle. And, of course, you may prefer to take your nitroglycerin in the form of a spray under the tongue.

Alpha-lipoic acid and diabetes. *Polyneuropathy*—numbness, pain, tingling of the extremities—is a common and difficult-to-treat complication of long-standing diabetes. According to new research, a daily dose of 600 milligrams of the antioxidant alpha-lipoic acid improved these symptoms after 3 weeks in more than half the patients treated.

Drink to prevent diabetes. Diabetes can be prevented in men and women by drinking four or more cups of coffee a day, mainly because of the caffeine. However other ingredients in the brew may play a part as well, since decaffeinated coffee also works (but to a lesser extent). Moderate intake of beer and wine also cuts the risk of diabetes, but only in women. However, heavy drinkers have a greater incidence of the disease.

Don't just sit there. Do something! Couples who have had trouble conceiving have heretofore been advised to reduce the frequency of their sexual activity so more sperm can accumulate. It turns out that's the wrong thing to do. Recent research indicates that such couples should try to have intercourse every 1 to 2 days. Doing so less frequently allows the sperm to accumulate and age within the genital areas and lose their potency. Fresh sperm are more likely to fertilize the egg. In the same vein, for women who have previously had a stillbirth or who have had a child and want another, the length of time between pregnancies is important. It always seems logical to wait. That's apparently wrong. According to new research, the longer you wait to become pregnant again, the greater the risk of stillbirth.

Cut the cost of Lipitor in half! The cost of drugs in the United States is prohibitive and often beyond the financial ability of many patients, especially those who are retired and on a fixed income. Changes in Medicare may not become effective for at least 2 years. Recent research indicates that at least for Lipitor (atorvastatin), one of the most commonly used drugs to lower cholesterol levels, taking the pill every other day instead of daily has the same effect on blood levels. Check with your doctor to see whether this applies to other members of the statin family of medications.

New drug adds height. In the past 16 years, growth hormone has been administered to 200,000 children worldwide who were extremely short because they had growth-stunting disease or their bodies were not producing enough growth hormone. The FDA has agonized for years whether this hormone should be given to more of these short children. Now, it has finally approved the administration of growth hormone somatropin (Humatrope, made by the Eli Lilly Company) when growth patterns suggest that a boy will not be taller than 5 feet 3 inches and a girl no more than 4 feet 11 inches. In such cases you can expect an additional 1.5 to 2.8 inches. When considering its use for your children, you should know that Humatrope must be injected six times a week for several years and costs between $10,000 and $25,000 a year. What's more, it is only available at selected drug stores, and can be prescribed only by designated specialists.

INDEX